All You Wanted to Know About Your Spine

A complete Guide to the Diagnosis and Alternative Treatment

Dr. Rahul K. Singh

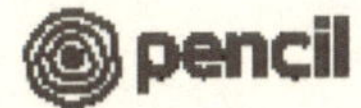

ISBN 978-93-5458-444-2

Published in India 2021 by Pencil

A brand of
One Point Six Technologies Pvt. Ltd.
123, Building J2, Shram Seva Premises,
Wadala Truck Terminal, Wadala (E)
Mumbai 400037, Maharashtra, INDIA
E connect@thepencilapp.com
W www.thepencilapp.com

Author biography

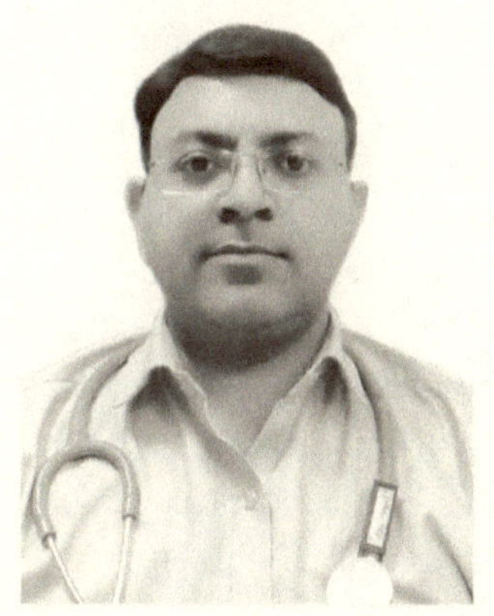

Dr. Rahul K. Singh is a registered homeopathic physician and a graduate of the "Bharati Vidyapeeth Homoeopathic Medical College", Pune, and post-graduated from the British Institute of Homoeopathy, London. He is practicing homeopathy since 2005 in Delhi and also working as a senior medical advisor in "Bhargava Phytolab Pvt. Ltd." (Oldest homoeopathic drugs manufacturer in INDIA), where he has been formulated many new homeopathic combination medicines including "AGUE NIL" syrup, a well-known homoeopathic medicine for the management of Dengue fever.

His achievements have been recognized by different awards, including the Chikitsa Seva Ratan Award (2020) by Akhil Bhartiya Chikitsak Association, Lifetime achievement award (2019) by Delhi Homoeopathic Federation, Special appreciation award (2018), Appreciation award (2017), and Dr. Hahnemann award (2016) by Board of Homoeopathic System of Medicine, Delhi and Safe hand award (2016) by Dr. Lal Foundation, etc.

Dr. Rahul has a good experience in R&D. He has involved in conducting many 'clinical trials' of homoeopathic medicines. Recently, he had successfully conducted a clinical trial on a homoeopathic combination for 'efficacy of homoeopathic combination syrup in Covid-19 patients', conducted at NIMS hospital, Jaipur. He was also the primary investigator (P.I) in this study.

His cured cases and write-ups have been published in different National and International journals and magazines. In addition to the clinical practice, he also organizes free health check-up camps individually or in association with different NGOs for the needy and poor patients. He is more specialized in treating Skin disorders, G.I.T. disorders, Endocrine disorders, Sexual problems, and Infertility.

CONTENTS

Foreword

It gives me immense pleasure in writing the foreword for this book on "Spinal Disorders and its Management" by Dr. Rahul Kumar Singh.

Having known Dr. Rahul Singh for about two decades, I have always admired his empathetic attitude towards patients. I find this book a culmination of his continuous efforts towards alleviating patient's sufferings.

In this book, the author has explained the diseases of spine and its homoeopathic treatment in such a nice manner that this book will prove to be of great help for students and practitioners both.

Today, diseases of spine have become a major medical problem. It also has considerable social and economic impact on the life of patients. This highlights the need for such a book which tells us how homoeopathic medicines can be a better way in managing these diseases. In my practice, I have many a times found patients having a perception that a "spinal disorder" necessarily means one is destined for lifelong pain and suffering. I am happy to find that through this book Dr. Rahul Singh has successfully broken this myth and has established the fact that homoeopathy is the best answer to such conditions.

I am confident that this book is going to be a great success. I congratulate the author for this endeavour and wish to see more and more such contributions from him in future.

Dr. Monika Srivastava
BHMS, MD, PhD(scholar)
Homoeopathic Medical Officer

Preface

I have been practicing homoeopathy for over 17 years. After watching so many patients for different ailments including acute and chronic ones, I realized that joints and back pain is the major reason for disability and agony in most of the patients. This world is full of suffering and we as a doctor can provide different treatment strategies that could be used to help the ailing population. I decided to write this book to describe the different disorders related to the spine and their management by yoga, diet, and homoeopathy to help the patients and other health professionals for better understanding.

Back pain is the commonest reason for absence from work and for seeking medical treatment. It can be uncomfortable and debilitating. Every movement seems to make it worse. It can result from injury, activity and some medical conditions. Back pain can affect people of any age, for different reasons. As people get older, the chance of developing lower back pain increases, due to factors such as previous occupation and degenerative disk disease.

Due to the anatomy of the spine, the description of the location of the back problems are very confusing for patients, and even for health care professionals who deal with back problems on a regular basis. Patients with back problems are all too often confused about what is pinching where, and how the back problem relates to their symptoms. Even when spine specialists spend a great deal of time explaining the problem, it is still often hard to understand. This is a common problem that is difficult to describe and difficult to understand. This book discusses how terminology used for spinal anatomy relates to common diagnoses and sources of back problems for patients.

The purpose of presenting this book is to compile all the disorders related to the spine at one point for a better understanding of the readers. In this book, I have tried to explain all the disorders related to the spine, their cause, risk factor, symptoms, diagnosis, and suggestive treatment. This book is for everyone who's struggling to get rid of the back problem and other disorders related to the spine. This book will explain the natural treatment methods and best practices to manage the different spinal disorders. The book also highlights the importance of physical exercise, yoga/asana and diet & regimen in managing Spinal disorders. It also elaborates the role of homoeopathy in treating spinal disorders.

This book is divided into ten chapters. The first chapter describes the functions of the spine, the anatomy of the spine, different parts contributing to the structure of the spine and their individual functions.

The second chapter deals with the history of spinal disorders, spinal injuries, and different spine problems, types of spinal curvatures, their causes, symptoms and their diagnosis.

The third chapter describes different types of spondylopathies including inflammatory and non-inflammatory. It also describes the pott's disease.

In the fourth chapter, intervertebral disc disorders have been described including Schmorl's nodes, Degenerative disc diseases, and Spinal disc herniation.

The fifth chapter deals with the pains related to spinal disorders like Sciatica pain and different radiculopathies.

Sixth chapter talks about different diagnostic test performed to diagnose the spinal disorders like History & physical examination of patient, different laboratory investigation for rule out any infection, X-ray, Myelogram, Magnetic resonance imaging (MRI), Computed tomography (CT scan), Nerve conduction velocity (NCV), Electromyography (EMG) and Spinal tap etc.

The seventh chapter is dedicated to different poses of yoga and asana for spinal health. Yoga is a natural and side-effect free remedy for Spinal disorders. Regular practice of yoga and different asana leads to a flexible body, calm mind and a positive attitude towards life.

The eighth chapter suggests some tips to keep your spine healthy and fit. It describes about the right posture during sitting, to take precaution during bending and lifting, importance of water intake, importance of exercise, rest and sound sleep for maintaining the health of spine and back.

In the ninth chapter, the importance of diet and nutrition for spine health is described. The importance of calcium diet and sources of dietary calcium is also discussed in this chapter.

The tenth chapter is dedicated to the role of

homoeopathy in different spinal disorders. Homoeopathic medicines are equally effective in acute as well as chronic conditions of spine disorders. In some conditions where reversal of disease is not possible, homoeopathy manages the complications of the particular problem and prevents further damage to joints and maintains the wellbeing of the patient without any harmful effects on the body. In this section, indicated symptoms of medicines have mentioned along with modalities to give a ready reference for the selection of remedy.

The Eleventh chapter includes the short repertory for quick reference.

This book does not set out to compete with the standard books on orthopedics and surgery neither it is an alternative to any other book related to the treatment of spine disorders. This is also not a homoeopathic 'Materia Medica'. My main purpose to compile this book is to give a basic understanding of spine disorders. The book highlights the importance of alternative therapies in spine disorders. It describes the role of yoga/asana, diet, and homoeopathy as an adjuvant with a basic treatment plan.

Dr. Rahul Kumar Singh
BHMS (Pune), HMD (London), CNCC

Acknowledgements

Writing a book is harder than I thought and more rewarding than I could have ever imagined. None of this would have been possible without the support of my wife, Jyoti. She stood by me during every struggle and all my successes.

I want to give special thanks to Late Dr. Pankaj Bhatnagar, who made me realized that homoeopathy is the best medical science and I can be a good homoeopath. I learned a lot of things from him, especially the confidence, I gained from working with him. Recently, he left for heavenly abode. His gentle soul will always be in my heart.

My sincere thanks also go to Mr. R.S. Bhargava, MD of Bhargava Phytolab Pvt. Ltd., for offering me the opportunity to work in his organization where I learned so many things related to homoeopathy and overall improved myself as a person. Here I met many good persons who influenced my life and encouraged me to do new things.

I also would like to thank you to my beloved wife, my family and relatives for supporting me throughout the years.

Finally, to all those who have been a part of my getting there: All my teachers, my friends and everyone who ever said anything positive to me or taught me something. I heard it all, and it meant something.

I am also thankful to my friends Dr. Monika Srivastava and Dr. Deepa Rajenimbalkar for encouraging me to write this book.

Last but not least; I want to thank my parents and God because without them I wouldn't be able to do any of this.

Dr. Rahul Kumar Singh

BHMS (Pune), HMD (London), CNCC

Introduction

The word "orthopaedic", is made up from two different greek words, "orthos", meaning straight, and "paidion", meaning child. The word "orthopaedic" is first used by a French pediatrician "Nicholas Andry" (1658-1742), who is also considered as the 'Father of Orthopedics.' The term orthopedic was used for the first time in the epoch-making textbook of Andry published in 1741.

Back pain is one of the commonest reasons for missed work. In fact, after upper respiratory infections, back pain is the second most common reason for visits to the doctors. It is estimated that one billion people worldwide are suffering from back pain. It affects all age groups, from children to the elderly. Back pain may be caused by muscle spasms, tense muscles, disc degeneration or disc herniation. To raise awareness of back pain and other spinal disorders, we celebrate 'World Spine Day' every year, on October 16. 'World Spine Day' highlights the importance of spinal health and wellbeing.

The Spine is a complicated structure of small bones, joints, ligaments and muscles. Due to flexibility of spine, you can sprain ligaments, strain muscles, rupture disks, and irritate joints, all of which can lead to back pain. Accidents and sports injuries can leads to severe back pain. Sometimes the simplest of movements like bending, to picking up something from the floor, can produce back pain. In addition, obesity, wrong or poor posture, joints diseases like arthritis and mental & physical stress can also cause or complicate back pain.

This book is going to solve all your queries related to disorders of spine, their management and treatment with diet & regimen, Yoga and Homoeopathy. With the help of health professionals, exercise and rehabilitation experts, we can prevent as well as manage most of the spine related disorders.

Homeopathy is the only form of treatment that has shown an overwhelming positive response in treating Spinal Disorders. Homeopathic medicines treat the person by the strengthening our vital force and provides protection from illness. Because of this personalized constitutional approach of homeopathy, a remedy that matches all of the symptoms of patients will stimulate vital force to revive balance and health.

Homoeopathy helps by stopping the demineralization and degeneration process of the bones of the joint involved. Homoeopathic remedies helps to Provide strength to the adjoining ligaments thus strengthening the whole joint, maintaining its space and decreasing pressure on the nerves. It may prevent fusion of joints and the further spread of disease in other organs. In mild and moderate disease stages complete cure has been achieved, in cases were the disease process has led to destruction of the joint as in severe cases homoeopathy can offer excellent palliative treatment without any side effects.

This book highlights the importance of alternative therapies in spine related disorders. Why diet

& regimen is important for spine health? Why yoga/asana is beneficial in managing the back pain and other spine disorders? This book will also explain the link between the spine disease and faulty life style. This book will acknowledge the efficacy of homoeopathic medicine in spine disorders and back pains.

Dr. Rahul Kumar Singh
BHMS (Pune), HMD (London), CNCC
Medical advisor: Bhargava Phytolab Pvt. Ltd.
Clinic: 182, Main Road Manadwali, near Badi Masjid,
Delhi – 110092
Contact: +91-9911167389
E-mail: drsingh_29@rediff.com,
drsingh67389@gmail.com

CHAPTER 1

KNOW YOUR SPINE

The origin of word spine drive from the Latin word "*Spina*"meaning backbone. Spine is one of the most important parts of our body. It gives structure and support to our body. Without Spine we could not stand up or keep ourselves upright. Spine provides the flexibility to move about freely and to bend with flexibility. The spine is also designed to protect our spinal cord. The spinal cord is a column of nerves that connects the brain to the rest of our body, allowing body to control its movements. One can't move any part of his body without the help of a spinal cord.

1.1 Functions of the Spine

- **Strength and Support -** Spine gives strength to the body and it also provides the support to the heavy weight of the skull. Cervical region support the skull, Thoracic region offers strength and stability to the middle part of body. Lumbar region carry the most of body's weight and allows movements. With the help of muscles, ligament and tendon, spine distribute body's weight.

- **Movement** - Special design of spine and its accompanying structures like muscles, tendons, ligaments and so forth, enable the body to move in various ways, for example, bowing, extending, turning and inclining.

- **Protection of Nerves** - Spinal column provides protection to the delicate nerves and the spinal cord, which helps to control the functions of our body. Vertebrae, muscles and ligaments attached to spine, form a network of protection that keeps the spinal cord from getting injured.

- **Blood Supply** - The vertebral bones of spine produce lot of red blood cells and minerals from its bone marrow. There are two types of bone marrow; red and yellow. Red bone marrow is responsible for the production of red blood cells, platelets and white blood cells, while yellow bone marrow contains high levels of fat cells and also produces some amounts of white blood cells.

- **Protection of Major Organs** - Thoracic vertebrae provides a base for the ribs to attach posteriorly while interiorly these are attached with sternum, which form a cage (ribcage) and protect our major organs like lungs and heart.

- **Absorption of Impact** - The spine acts as a shock absorber, and absorbs the impact with the help of inter-vertebral discs. These discs are situated between each vertebra and prevents the vertebrae from 'knocking' into each other.

1.2 Anatomy of Spine

The spine is also called as vertebral column which is made up of 33 bones, called vertebrae. The upper 24 are articulating and separated from each other by inter-vertebral discs, and the lower nine are fused, 5 in the sacrum and 4 in the coccyx or tailbone. The name of articulating vertebras is kept according to their presence in the region of the spine.

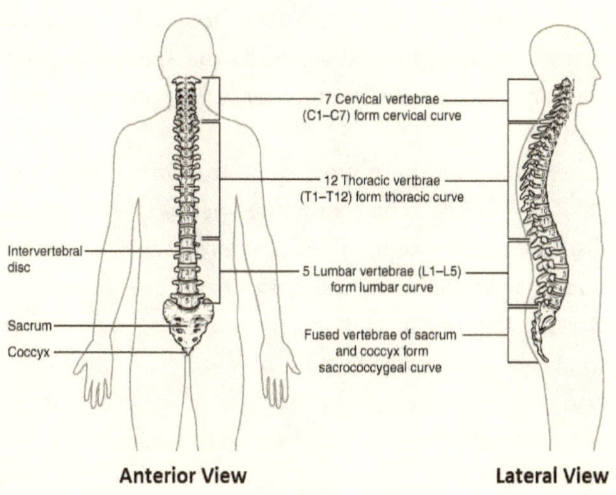

Figure 1.1: Anatomy of Spine

- **First Seven – Cervical (C1 to C7) – at nape of neck**

- **Next Twelve – Thoracic (T1 to T12) – at back of chest**
- **Next Five – Lumber (L1 to L5) – at lower back**
- **Next Five – Sacral S1 to S5 (Fused) – at pelvis**
- **Last Four – Coccyx (Fused) – above anus**

Ligaments and muscles associate these bones together to shape the spinal column. The spinal column gives the body structure and function. The spinal column holds and protects the spinal cord, which is a bundle of nerves that sends signals to other parts of the body. There are so many muscles which attached to the spine and provide support the upright posture of the spine and help to move the spine.

When you look the normal spine from the side, it has an "S"-like curve. This structure permits for an even distribution of weight. The "S" curve enables a healthy & normal spine to withstand a wider range of pressure and stress. Despite the fact that the lower segment of your spine holds the greater part of the body's weight, each portion depends upon the strength of the others to work appropriately.

1.2.1 Cervical Spine (Neck)

The Cervical Spine is comprised of the initial 7 vertebrae in the spine. It begins just underneath the skull and finishes just above the thoracic spine. The cervical spine has a lordotic curve, a backward "C"-shape-just like the lumbar spine. The cervical spine is substantially more portable than other spinal regions.

In contrast to other region of the spine, there are special openings in every vertebra in the cervical spine for arteries. These arteries bring blood to the brain.

Two vertebrae in the cervical spine, the atlas and the axis, differ from the other vertebrae because they are designed specifically for rotation.

The atlas sits on top of the second cervical vertebra, the axis. Special ligaments between the atlas and the axis allow for a great deal of rotation. It is this special arrangement that allows the head to move in so many directions.

1.2.2 Thoracic Spine (Mid Back)

The thoracic spine is comprised of the middle 12 vertebrae. These vertebrae connect to your ribs and form part of the back wall of the thorax. The thoracic spine's curve is kyphotic, a "C"-shaped curve with the opening of the "C" in the front. Inter-vertebral discs of this part of the spine are very narrow and thin. Rib connections and thin discs in the thoracic spine limit the free movement of the spine in the mid back in comparison to the lumbar or cervical parts of the spine. Also, the space inside the spinal canal is very less.

1.2.3 Lumbar Spine (Low Back)

The lowest part of the spine is known as the lumbar spine. Usually, Lumbar region is comprised of 5 vertebrae. However, sometimes people are born with a

sixth vertebra in the lumbar region.
The lumbar spine's shape has a lordotic curve-shaped like a backward "C". The vertebrae in the lumbar spine area are the largest of the entire spine. The lumbar spinal canal is also larger than in the cervical or thoracic parts of the spine. The size of the lumbar spine allows for more space for nerves to move about.

1.2.4 Sacrum and coccyx or tailbone

These are fused bone and make a part of sacrum.

1.3 Important Structures of the Spine

- Vertebrae
- Inter-vertebral Discs
- Facet Joints
- Neural Foraminae
- Spinal Cord
- Nerve Roots
- Paraspinal Muscles
- Spinal Segments

1.3.1 Vertebrae

The word vertebra derives from the Latin word "vertebra", which is related to the Latin verb "vertere" meaning "to turn". The great anatomist Andreas Vesalius (1514-1564) finally introduces the word "vertebra" as an anatomical term.
Spine is made up of 33 small bones, called vertebrae. The vertebrae protect and support the spinal cord. They also bear the majority of the weight put upon your spine.

1.3.2 Inter-vertebral Disc

There is a soft, gel-like cushion between each vertebra, which is called an intervertebral disc. These flat & round "cushions" act like shock absorbers by helping absorb pressure. The discs prevent the bones from rubbing against each other.

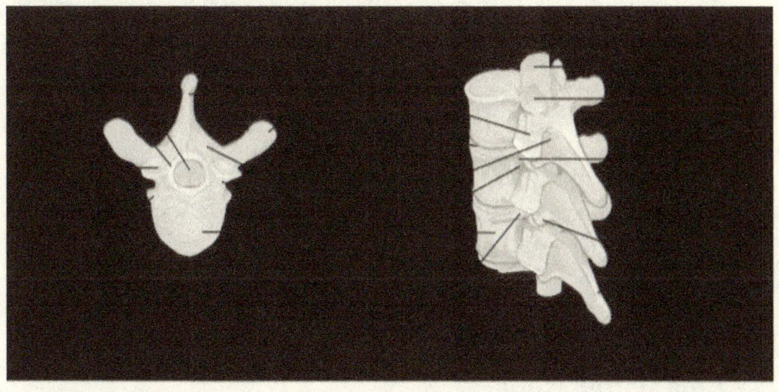

Figure 1.2: Some important structures of the spine

1.3.3 Facet Joints

Just like knee and elbow joints, spinal column also has real joints which are called facet joints. The facet joints connect the vertebrae together and give them the flexibility to move against each other. There are two facet joints between each pair of vertebrae, one on each side.

1.3.4 Neural Foramina

The spinal cord branches off into 31 pairs of nerve roots, which exit the spine through small openings on each side of the vertebra called neural foramina. The two nerve roots in each pair go in opposite directions when traveling through the foramina. One goes out the left foramina; the other goes out through the right foramina. The nerve root allows nerve signals to travel to and from your brain to the rest of your body.

1.3.5 Spinal Cord

The spinal cord is a bundle of millions of nerve fibers that carries messages from your brain to the rest of the body. It starts from the brain and end to the area between the end of our first lumbar vertebra and top of the second lumbar vertebra. Each vertebra has a hole in the center, so when they stack on top of each other they form a hollow tube (spinal canal) that holds and protects the entire spinal cord and its nerve roots.

1.3.6 Nerve Roots

The nerve fibers in your spinal cord branch off to form pairs of nerve roots that travel through the small openings between the vertebrae. The nerves in each area of the spinal cord connect to specific parts of our body. This is why damage to the spinal cord can cause paralysis in certain areas and not others. It depends on which spinal nerves are affected.

1.3.7 Paraspinal Muscles

The muscles next to the spine are called the paraspinal muscles. They support the spine and provide the motor for movement of the spine. Joints allow flexibility, and muscles allow mobility. There are many small muscles in the back. Each controls some part of the total movement between the vertebrae and the rest of the skeleton.

1.3.8 Spinal Segments

A spinal segment is made up of two vertebrae attached together by ligaments, with a soft disc separating them. The facet joints fit between the two vertebrae, allowing for movement, and the neural foramina between the vertebrae allow space for the nerve roots to travel freely from the spinal cord to the body. The spinal segment allows physicians to examine the repeating parts of the spinal column to understand what can go wrong with the various parts of the spine.

CHAPTER 2

SPINAL INJURIES AND DISORDERS

2.1 History of Spinal disorders

History of spinal deformities begins in ancient Greece. What we know today for diagnosis and management of spinal deformities/disorders are a summarization of study of spine in ancient Greece, mainly from the medical treatises of Hippocrates and Galen. Hippocrates, through precise perception and intelligent thinking was led to accurate conclusions firstly for the structure of the spine and secondly for its diseases. He introduced the terms kyphosis and scoliosis and wrote in depth about diagnosis and treatment of kyphosis and less about scoliosis. Nearly five centuries later, Galen, impressively described scoliosis, lordosis and kyphosis, provided aetiologic implications and used the same principles with Hippocrates for their management, while his studies influenced therapeutic practice on spinal deformations for over 1500 years.

2.2 Spinal Injuries and Disorders

Spinal Injuries or Spinal cord injury (SCI) is a devastating neurological injury, resulting in varying degrees of paralysis, sensory loss and sphincter disturbance which are permanent and irreversible in cases. It was labeled as "an ailment not to be treated" in the Edwin Smith papyrus 5000 years ago (Feldman and Goodrich 1999). Unfortunately, very little has changed, in many parts of the world like in underdeveloped countries. SCI has been studied in detail in the Developed world, and thousands of manuscripts have been published in the last few decades. These include large scale epidemiologic surveys, multicenter research on interventions in acute SCI, reports on complications from acute and chronic SCI, results of rehabilitation interventions and functional outcomes. But all this covers only a part of the world population.

Spinal disorders are among the most widely recognized ailments with critical effect on health related quality of life. Various spinal disorders and conditions can affect the vertebrae, inter-vertebral discs and ligaments, thereby diminishing the functions of the spinal column. Degenerative disc disease, osteophytes, foraminal stenosis and herniated discs are some of the more debilitating conditions which can lead to pain, numbness, tingling, spasms and muscle weakness. Pain is the major symptoms of Spinal injuries and disorders.

To understand Spinal deformities, we can divide spinal disorders according to their pathology.

Spinal Disorders/Dorsopathies		
DEFORMING DORSOPATHIES	**Spinal curvature**	**Kyphosis**
		Scoliosis
		Lordosis
	Other	**Scheuermann's disease**
		Torticollis
SPONDYLOPATHY	**Inflammatory**	**Spondylitis**
		Ankylosing spondylitis
		Sacroiliitis
		Discitis
		Spondylodiscitis
		Pott disease
	Non-inflammatory	**Spondylosis**
		Spondylolysis
		Spondylolisthesis
		Spinal stenosis
		Facet syndrome
INTER-VERTEBRAL DISC DISORDER		**Schmorl's nodes**
		Degenerative disc disease
		Spinal disc herniation
BACK PAIN		**Neck pain**
		Upper back pain
		Low back pain
		Coccydynia
		Sciatica
		Radiculopathy

Figure 2.1: Different types of dorsopathies

2.3 Deforming Dorsopathies

Dorsopathies refers to the conditions impairing the backbone. These include various diseases of the back or spine such as spinal curvature disorders.

2.3.1 Spinal curvature

A healthy spine when viewed from the side has gentle curves to it. The curves help the spine absorb stress from body movement and gravity.
When viewed from the back, the spine should run straight down the middle of the back. When abnormalities of the spine occur, the natural curvatures of the spine are misaligned or exaggerated in certain areas.

2.3.2 Types of spine curvature disorders

Spine curvature disorders are the disorders which are caused by dislocation, degeneration or injury to any of the vertebrae from spine. Old people, mainly the men above 65 years are commonly affected by these disorders. There are three main types of spine curvature disorders, including kyphosis, lordosis and scoliosis.

2.3.2.1 Kyphosis

The word Kyphosis is derived from the Greek word "Kyphos" meaning "hunchback" or "bent". Kyphosis is characterized by an abnormally rounded upper back (more than 50 degrees of curvature).

2.3.2.2 Lordosis

The term Lordosis is also belong to the Greek word "lordos" meaning " forward curving" Also called swayback, the spine of a person with lordosis curves significantly inward at the lower back.

2.3.2.3 Scoliosis

The term scoliosis is also derived from the Greek word "scolios" meaning 'curvature' and was coined by the Greek physician Galen of Pergamon (130-200 A.D). A person with scoliosis has a sideways curve to their spine. The curve is often S-shaped or C-shaped.

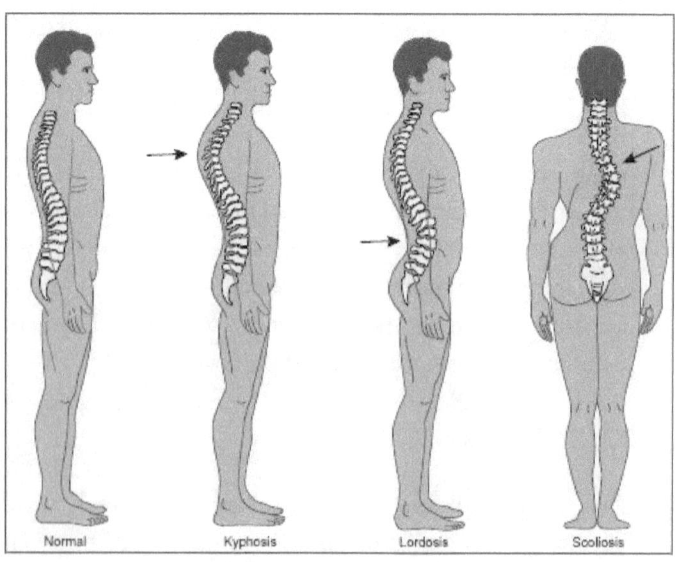

Figure 2.2: Different types of spine curvature disorders

2.3.3 Causes of spine curvature disorders

A. Causes for lordosis

- Achondroplasia - A disorder in which bones do not grow normally, resulting dwarfism
- Spondylolisthesis - A condition in which a vertebra, slips forward
- Osteoporosis
- Obesity
- Kyphosis - A condition marked by an abnormally rounded upper back
- Discitis - Inflammation of the disc space between the bones of the spine
- Benign (harmless) juvenile lordosis

B. Cause for kyphosis

- Abnormal vertebrae development in-utero (congenital kyphosis)
- Poor posture
- Scheuermann's disease - A condition that causes vertebrae to be misshaped
- Arthritis
- Osteoporosis

- Spina bifida - A birth defect in which the spinal column of the fetus does not close completely during development inside the womb

- Spine infections or Spine tumors

C. Causes of scoliosis

- Neuromuscular conditions - These affect the nerves and muscles and include cerebral palsy and muscular dystrophy

- Congenital scoliosis (present at birth) - This is rare condition and occurs because the bones in the spine developed abnormally when the fetus was growing inside the mother

- Genes - At least one gene is thought to be involved in scoliosis

- Leg length - If one leg is longer than the other, the individual may develop scoliosis

- Other causes - Bad posture, carrying backpacks or satchels, and some injuries

2.3.4 Symptoms of spine curvature disorders

A. Symptoms of lordosis may include

- Appearing swayback, with the buttocks being more pronounced

- Having a large gap between the lower back and the floor when lying on your back on a hard surface that does not change when you bend forward

- Back pain and discomfort

- Problems moving certain ways

B. Symptoms of kyphosis are usually visible in nature and include

- Bending forward of the head compared to the rest of the body

- Hump or curve to the upper back

- Fatigue in back or legs

- Postural kyphosis does not typically cause back pain; however, physical activity and long periods of standing and sitting can cause discomfort for people with Scheuermann's kyphosis

C. Symptoms of scoliosis may include having

- Uneven shoulder blades with one being higher than the other

- An uneven waist or hip

- Leaning toward one side

2.3.5 Treatment of spinal curvature disorders

In general, treatment is determined based on the severity and type of spinal curvature disorder you have. Mild spinal curvature, as occurs with postural kyphosis, may not be treated at all. More severe spinal curvature may require the use of a back brace or surgery.

A. Treatment for lordosis may include

- Medication to relieve pain and swelling
- Exercise and physical therapy to increase muscle strength and flexibility
- Wearing a back brace
- Weight loss
- Surgery

B. Treatment for kyphosis may include

- Exercise and anti-inflammatory medication to ease pain or discomfort
- Wearing a back brace
- Surgery to correct severe spine curvature and congenital kyphosis
- Exercises and physical therapy to increase muscle strength

C. Treatment for scoliosis may include

- **Observation** -If there is a slight curve your doctor may choose to check your back every four to six months to see if the curve gets worse

- **Bracing** -Depending on the degree of the curve, a back brace is sometimes prescribed for kids and adolescents who are still growing. Bracing can help prevent the curve from getting worse

- **Surgery** -If the curve is severe and is getting worse, surgery is sometimes needed

Exercise programs, chiropractic treatment, electrical stimulation, and nutritional supplements have not been proven to prevent the worsening of scoliosis. It is still ideal to keep as much as strength and flexibility to maintain normal function. This may require more effort and attention in someone with scoliosis.

2.3.6 Others

Deforming dorsopathies other than disorders of spinal curvature comes under this category.

2.3.6.1 Scheuermann's disease

Scheuermann's disease (also known as juvenile kyphosis, as it is mostly found in teenagers) is a self-limiting skeletal deformity in the thoracic or thoraco-lumbar spine in which pediatric patients have an increased kyphosis along with backache and localized changes in the vertebral bodies. It is named after 'Holger Werfel Scheuermann', a Danish surgeon.

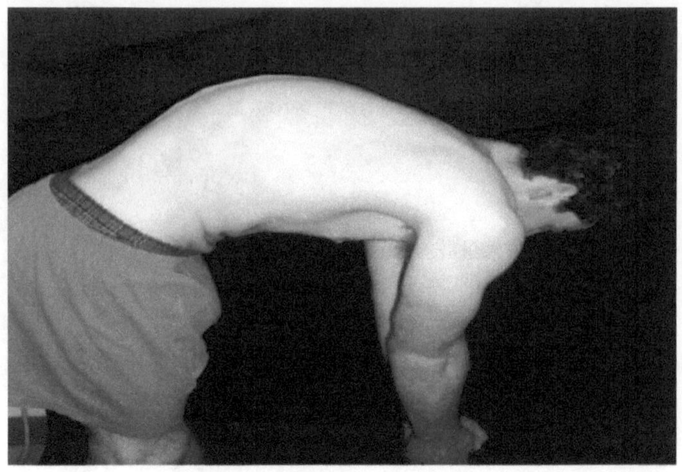

Figure 2.3: Scheuermann's disease

In Scheuermann's disease, the vertebrae grow unevenly with respect to the sagittal plane; that means, the posterior angle is often greater than the anterior. This uneven growth of vertebrae gives a "wedging" shape, causing kyphosis.

Symptoms:

Scheuermann's disease is mostly found in teenagers and presents a deformity worse than postural kyphosis. Symptoms includes-

- Tiredness and muscle stiffness, especially after a day of sitting in class
- Limited flexibility
- Muscular cramps and spasms

- Pain in and around the thoracic spine which become worse by sports activities like twisting, bending and arching etc
- Restriction in range of movement especially into extension (bending backwards)
- It leads to an increased thoracic or mid/upper back kyphosis (bend)
- Patient rarely get any Serious damage but it is possible in case of pressure effects on spinal cord or nearby organ such as lungs

Cause:

Presently, the exact cause for Scheuermann's disease is unknown, and the condition gives off an impression of being multi-factorial. Several candidate genes (such as COL1A2, which has been related with Marfan syndrome) have been proposed and excluded.

Diagnosis:

Diagnosis is based on physical examination of patient and by medical imaging. X-rays are the most valuable imaging test for diagnosing Scheuermann's disease.

Treatment:

Scheuermann's diseases is considered as self-limiting disease and many a times, no treatment is required. In some cases where patient is having pain or problem in flexibility, treatment may require. Restoration of muscles movement is also required for getting relief. Treatment plan may follow -

- Medication like NSAID to relieve pain and swelling
- Inflammation can be reduced by ice therapy, exercise and physical therapy
- Physiotherapy, electrotherapy, acupuncture can be used to increase muscle strength and flexibility
- Surgery is rarely required but may needed in case of severe deformity or for cosmetic reasons

2.3.6.2 Torticollis

The term Torticollis is derived from the Latin words 'tortus' for twisted and 'collum' for neck. The neck tends to twist to one side while chin tilts to the other side, causing head tilt.

Torticollis, also known as wry neck or loxia, is one of a more extensive classification of disorder defined by an abnormal, asymmetrical head or neck position. It exhibits flexion, extension, or twisting of muscles of the neck beyond their normal position.

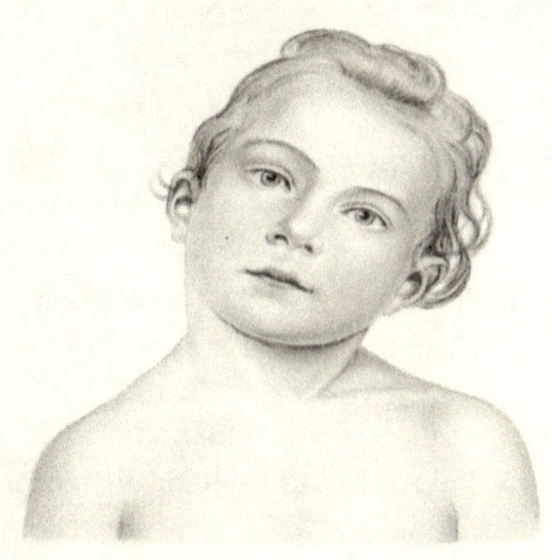

Figure 2.4: Torticollis

Causes

This condition can be congenital or acquired. It can also be developed in the womb due to wrong position of baby's head. A damage in neck muscles or lack of blood supply can also lead to the wry neck. Injury to neck and spine or any infection of the head & neck are some other causes.

Types of torticollis

- **Congenital muscular torticollis** -The cause of congenital muscular torticollis is unclear. Birth trauma or intrauterine malposition is considered to be the cause of damage to the sternocleidomastoid muscle in the neck.

- **Acquired -**It may develop as a result from disease of cervical vertebrae, adenitis, tonsillitis, rheumatism, enlarged cervical glands, retropharyngeal abscess, or damage to the nervous system, upper spine, or muscles. It may be spasmodic (clonic) or permanent (tonic). The permanent type may be due to Pott's disease (tuberculosis of the spine).

- **Idiopathic -** If the condition occurs without a known cause, it is called idiopathic torticollis.

Symptoms of torticollis

Symptoms of torticollis may vary from person to person. Physical appearance of tilted neck is the most apparent sign & symptom.

- Limited scope of movement of the head
- Headache
- Head tremor
- Pain & Stiffness of the neck muscles
- One shoulder is higher than the other
- Swelling of the neck muscles (possibly present at birth)
- The head tilts to one side while the chin tilts to the other -

1. Laterocollis - The head is tipped toward the shoulder
2. Rotational torticollis - The head rotates along the longitudal axis
3. Anterocollis - Forward flexion of the head and neck
4. Retrocollis - Hyperextension of head and neck backward

Diagnosis:

- By physical examination
- CT scan of the neck
- X-ray and MRI scan to find out the structural problem
- MRI of the brain
- Electromyogram (EMG) to see which muscles are most affected
- Blood tests to look for medical conditions that are linked to torticollis

Treatment of torticollis

As of now, there is no way to prevent wry neck. However, early inception of treatment is very important for full recovery and to decrease the chance of relapse. Following treatment options can work -

- Initially, the condition is treated with physical therapies, such as stretching to release tightness, strengthening exercises to improve muscular balance, and handling to stimulate symmetry

- Congenital forms of wry neck can be treated by stretching the neck muscles. If treatment started within a few months of birth, this can be very successful

- A TOT collars

- Neck braces

- Massage of affected area

- Heat therapy

- Medication – pain medicines, muscles relaxants, etc

- Surgery – if other treatments don't work, surgery can sometimes correct the problem

CHAPTER 3

SPONDYLOPATHY

Spondylopathy is a general term for disorders of the vertebrae. It is commonly associated with compression of peripheral nerve roots and spinal cord, causing pain and stiffness of the part. These can be:

3.1. Inflammatory Spondylopathy

- Spondy
- litis – Cervical & Lumbar
- Ankylosing spondylitis
- Sacroiliitis
- Discitis
- Spondylodiscitis
- Pott disease

3.2. Non-inflammatory

- Spondylosis
- Spondylolysis
- Spondylolisthesis
- Spinal
- Stenosis
- Facet syndrome

3.1.1 Spondylitis

Spondylitis is an inflammation of the vertebra. It is one of the most common causes of pain in neck and back. Spondylitis is a classification of several different inflammatory arthritic conditions that are not rheumatic and which primarily affect the spine. Spondylitis is a chronic condition characterized by inflammation of the joint capsules and ligaments.

Most common types of spondylitis are: -

- **Cervical spondylitis** - Inflammation of the bones and muscles of cervical spine (C1 – C7)
- **Ankylosing spondylitis** -It mainly affects the joints in the spine and the sacroiliac joint in the pelvis

- **Lumbar spondylitis -** Pain and inflammation of bones and muscles of lower spine (L1 – L5)

3.1.1.1 Cervical Spondylitis

When there is an inflammation of joints and muscles of cervical region, it is called Cervical Spondylitis. It also referred as arthritis of neck. As cervical region is most flexible part of the spine, so it is more vulnerable area to get injury.

Risk of injury to cervical region

In comparison to whole spine, the cervical spine is most flexible, so chances of injury are more in this region from any strong and sudden movements. This high risk of injury is due to the limited support to the muscles in the cervical area, while this part of the spine has to support the weight of the head-an average of 15 pounds. This is a lot of weight for a small, thin set of bones and soft tissues to bear. Sudden, strong head movements can cause damage to the joints and muscles of this region.

Causes of Cervical Spondylitis

- Stiffness in muscles of the cervical region for prolonged period (like driving for long distance without break), cause a kinking of the cervical spine to the front.
- Bad sitting posture or working for long on Computer.

- Lacks of exercise of the cervical region can cause weakness of the muscles of cervical spine.

- Using several pillows when lying at bed cause propping up the neck into an unnatural position which affect the alignment of the cervical column, causing a forward inclination.

- A job that requires heavy weight lifting or a lot of bending and twisting can cause injury to the cervical spine.

- Past neck injury (may be several years before).

Pathology

- Narrowing of the cervical vertebrae with the reduction of disc space.

- Formation of an osteophyte (bony spur) due to friction between two vertebral bodies created by this narrowing.

- Loss of normal concavity in the cervical region, i.e., loss of lordosis.

- Compression of the cervical nerve roots.

- Vascular insufficiency - The vertebro-basilar vessels are important arteries coursing along the cervical column to the back of the brain. There are areas here that serve balance and posture. If the blood flow is affected, the corresponding function is also affected. This syndrome is known as vertebro-basilar insufficiency. The problems of vascular insufficiency consist of vertigo, giddiness, occasional tinnitus, a sense of unsteadiness, etc. In a severe case, there is transient loss of consciousness.

Symptoms

- Pain in neck & shoulder
- Stiffness in the neck & shoulder, especially in the morning
- Neck pain due to movement of neck
- Radiating pain from neck to arms on both side and back of head
- Vertigo
- Headache
- Numbness and tingling sensation in the hands
- Weakness in hands
- May feel irritable, fatigue, disturb sleep and impair ability to work

Diagnosis

- Depends upon the symptoms described by the patient - like Pain, vertigo, uneasiness, stiffness, headache and tingling numbness in hands etc.

- Physical examination—by identifying the tender spots along the neck and testing the ability to move the neck in various directions in severe cases.

Investigations

- X-RAY of Cervical region
- C T Scan of Cervical Region
- MRI of Spine
- Nerve Function Tests - An electro-myogram (EMG) is used to check if the nerves are functioning normally or not.

Treatment

- Rest
- Painkillers
- Wearing a cervical collar to provide support to the neck and limit the movement
- Application of heat and cold therapy, traction, Physiotherapy or exercise
- Non-steroidal anti-inflammatory drugs (NSAIDs)
- A low-dose tricyclic antidepressant
- Surgery in extreme case

3.1.2 Ankylosing spondylitis

The word ankylosing spondylitis is originates form a greek derivation where 'ankylos' means - "bent", 'spondylos' means – "vertebra" and 'itis' means – "inflammation".

It is a chronic inflammatory disease of the axial skeleton, with variable involvement of peripheral joints and non-articular structures. It mainly affects joints in the spine and the sacroiliac joint in the pelvis. In severe cases, it can eventually cause complete fusion and rigidity of the spine (Bamboo Spine).

Bamboo Spine

Bamboo spine is a radiographic feature seen in ankylosing spondylitis that occurs as a result of vertebral body fusion by marginal syndesmophytes. "Bamboo spine" develops when the outer fibers of the fibrous ring of the inter-vertebral disks ossify, which results in the formation of marginal syndesmophytes between adjoining vertebrae.

A bamboo spine typically involves the thoraco-lumbar and or lumbo-sacral junctions and predisposes to unstable vertebral fractures and Andersson lesions.

There is also accompanying squaring of the anterior vertebral body margins with associated reactive sclerosis of the vertebral body margins (shiny corner sign). Together these give the impression of undulating continuous lateral spinal borders on AP spinal radiographs and resemble a bamboo stem; therefore it is termed as bamboo spine.

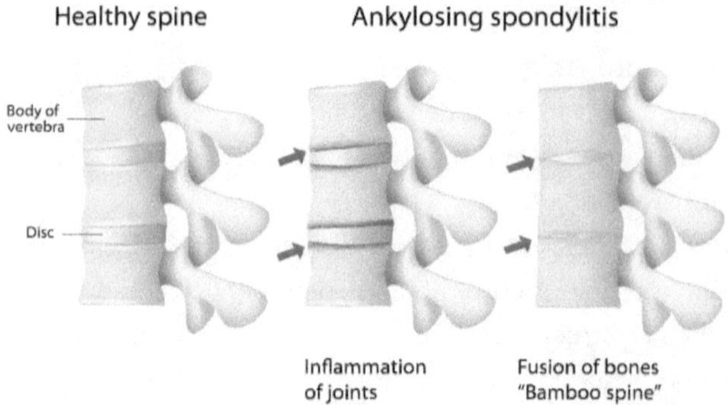

Figure 3.1: Ankylosing spondylitis and 'bamboo spine'

Pathophysiology

Ankylosing spondylitis (AS) is a systemic rheumatic disease, meaning it affects the entire body. Approximately 90% of AS patients express the HLA-B27 genotype, meaning there is a strong genetic association. It usually begins in the second or third decade of life and tends to occur more often in males.

Symptoms

The disease starts with low back pain that comes and goes. Low back pain is present most of the time as the condition progresses.

- Pain and stiffness are worse at night, in the morning, or when you are in rest. The discomfort may cause sleeplessness.

- Pain gets better by exercise or by some activity, most of the time.
- Usually, back pain begins in the sacroiliac joints (between the pelvis and spine). Over time, it may involve whole spine or some part of it.
- Flexibility of your lower spine become reduces. After some time, you may stand in a hunched forward position.

Other parts of your body that may be stiff and painful include:

- The joints between your ribs and breastbone or sternum, so that there is difficulty in fully expansion of chest.
- Pain & Swelling in the joints of the shoulders, knees and ankles.
- Swelling of the eye.
- Fatigue is also a common symptom.

Less common symptoms include:

- Loss of appetite
- Slight fever
- Weight loss

Complications of AS (Ankylosing spondylitis)

- Osteoporosis
- Quadriplegia
- Spinal fracture
- Cauda equina syndrome
- Spontaneous subluxation of the atlantoaxial joint
- Spondylodiscitis
- Amyloidosis
- Conjunctivitis
- Depigmentation and scarring of iris
- Acute iritis/ uveitis or Eye inflammation
- Cardiomegaly
- Pericarditis
- Mitral incompetence
- Cardiac conduction defects
- Aortic incompetence
- Apical pulmonary fibrosis with cavitation
- Prostatitis

- Glomerulonephritis

Exams and Tests

Tests may include:

- CBC including ESR (To measure the inflammation)
- HLA-B27 antigen (which detects the gene linked to ankylosing spondylitis)
- X-rays of the spine and pelvis
- MRI of the spine
- Measurements of the chest when breathing.

Treatment

As if now, there is no cure for ankylosing spondylitis (AS), however treatments and medications can diminish the manifestations like pain and other symptoms. The goals of treatment are to reduce pain and stiffness, maintain a good posture, prevent deformity, and preserve the ability to perform normal activities. Protein rich diet and vegetables are beneficial for patients with AS. In severe cases, surgery can be an option in the form of joint replacements.

3.1.3 Sacroiliitis

Sacroiliitis is an inflammation of one or both of sacroiliac joints. — The places where lower spine and pelvis connect. Sacroiliitis can cause pain in buttocks or lower back, and may even extend down one or both legs. The pain associated with sacroiliitis is often aggravated by prolonged standing or by stair climbing.

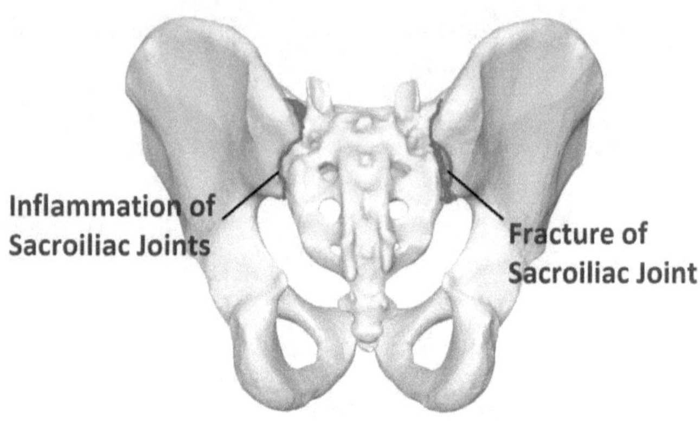

Figure 3.2: Sacroiliitis

Symptoms

The most common symptom is pain, which can affect the leg, groin and feet and can be aggravated by:

- Prolonged standing
- Bearing more weight on one leg than the other
- Stair climbing
- Running

Patient may have slight fever. Stiffness of hip & low back especially in morning and after sitting still for a long time.

Causes

There are many causes for sacroiliac joint dysfunction such as:

- **Traumatic injury -** A sudden impact, such as a motor vehicle accident or a fall, can damage sacroiliac joints.
- **Arthritis -** Arthritis or osteoarthritis can occur in sacroiliac joints and affects the spine.
- **Ankylosing spondylitis -**This is an inflammatory arthritis that affects the spine and hips. Sacroiliitis is considered as an early sign of this sacroiliitis. But it is not necessary that all people having sacroiliitis must have ankylosing spondylitis.
- **Pregnancy -** When a woman is pregnant, her sacroiliac joints stretch to make room for the growing baby. This may put stress on the joints and cause sacroiliitis.
- **Infection -** In rare cases, the sacroiliac joint can become infected.

Diagnosis

- Physical examination - To locate the site of pain or tenderness
- Blood tests - To find out any signs of inflammation
- X-ray - To find out any damage in sacroiliac joints
- MRI – For more advance findings

Treatment

Treatment of sacroiliitis depends on its types. Over the counter pain medications can be taken for pain relief. But in case of pregnancy, one should consult with their doctor before taking any medication. Treatment options for sacroiliitis include:

- Alternating ice and heat to relieve pain and inflammation
- Physical therapy and exercise
- **Medication –**NSAIDs or muscle relaxants to reduce pain and spasm. Tumor necrosis factor (TNF) inhibitors can be used to relieve the pain of sacroiliitis associated with ankylosing spondylitis or psoriatic arthritis.
- Injections of corticosteroids directly into the joint to reduce pain & inflammation

- **Surgery** -In rare cases, to fuse bone in joints together to relieve the pain

3.1.4 Discitis

Discitis or diskitis is an inflammation of the inter-vertebral disc space. It is typically a bacterial disease however might be viral. It will cause swelling in intervertebral disc space and can put pressure on the disc and thus pain.

It may affect any age groups, but usually affects children under 8 years of age. In any case, discitis occurs post surgically in approximately 1-2 percent of patients after spinal surgery.

Pathophysiology

Discitis is mainly a result of an infection. However, infection does not ordinarily begin in the vertebra or disk space; rather, it spreads there from different destinations through the circulatory system (hematogenous spread) to reach the spinal column. The blood supply to the spinal column is via the spinal arteries and to a lesser extent from the radicular arteries.

This hematogenous spread originates from a systemic infection, like urinary tract infection (UTI). Many sites of origin have been implicated, but UTI, pneumonia, and soft-tissue infection appear to be the most widely recognized. Intravenous (IV) drug use with contaminated syringes may cause direct access to the bloodstream for a variety of organisms. Often, no other site of infection is found.

Staphylococcus aureus is the organism most commonly

found; however, *Escherichia coli* and *Proteus* species are more common in patients with UTIs.

Signs and Symptoms

- Severe pain in lower back, which cause difficulty in mobility.
- Pain may also spread from the back to the other parts of the body like abdomen, hip, leg or groin.
- Frequent leaning of back.
- Difficulty while getting up from the floor.
- Mild fever with feeling of tiredness.
- Difficulty while raising the leg in the upward direction when lying down on the back.
- Children may refuse to walk due to severe pain.
- Loss of appetite.
- Sweating with sudden chills.

Causes

- Post-operatively - Due to the aftereffect of an intervention at the site of the infection by a surgical, diagnostic or therapeutic procedure. For instance, surgery on the back or a needle placed in the back for a diagnostic or treatment can introduce pathogens.

- Second is "spontaneous" discitis that is caused by an infecting organism, either bacteria or virus.

The more common bacteria include:

- Staphylococcus aureus
- Escherichia coli
- Pseudomonas aeruginosa
- Proteus species
- Klebsiella species

Risk factors

Any person can develop discitis but it is more likely in one or more of the following risk factors.

- Adults around 50 years
- Children under 10 years
- People suffering from Diabetes mellitus
- People having HIV infection / AIDS
- People having autoimmune disorders
- Long term steroid users
- Cancer patients, especially when on chemotherapy
- Patients suffering from Kidney failure

Diagnosis

On the basis of symptoms alone, Discitis is very difficult to diagnose. So, various other investigations are required to diagnose the discitis, such as:

- Blood tests - to find out the infection
- Sputum and urine test may require to find out the infection
- CT scan
- X-rays
- MRIs
- Biopsies

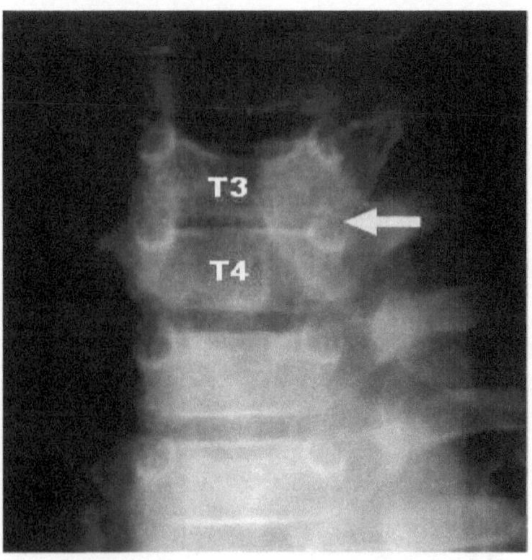

Figure 3.3: X-ray report of discitis

Treatment

Treatment includes medication to treat infections & pain and reduce the mobility:

- Antibiotics to combat infections
- Anti-inflammatory drugs to treat an auto immune reaction
- NSAIDs to relieve pain
- Changes in daily activities or bed rest in severe cases
- Reducing the mobility of the affected region, by using back brace or a plaster cast
- Surgical correction in case of abscess formation

3.1.5 Spondylodiscitis

As name suggests, spondylodiscitis is a combination of discitis and spondylitis. It can lead to osteomyelitis of the spinal column.
It is the most common complication of local infection or an abscess and is a rare but serious infection.

Cause

Staphylococci and Mycobacterium tuberculosis are the main causative organisms. Less common causative organisms are E. coli, fungi, Brucella spp. and zoonoses. Spondylodiscitis frequently develops in immuno-compromised individuals, such as by a cancer, infection, or by immunosuppressive drugs used for organ transplantations.

Types

It is basically of two types which are endogenous and exogenous.

- **Endogenous Spondylodiscitis** -The primary infection begins quite far away from the vertebral system and then the infection reaches the vertebral bodies through the blood. The inflammation then spreads to the ventral sections of spinal column.

- **Exogenous Spondylodiscitis** -The root cause may be some sort of surgical procedure or any injection to the vertebral column.

Symptoms of Spondylodiscitis

- Severe back pain

- Neck pain radiating to the chest or abdomen

- Some neurological symptoms like weakness of the legs, paralysis of the extremities, altered sensation may present

- Fever may present

- The most common symptom will be visible spine deformities like kyphosis

- Weight loss

Diagnosis

As Spondylodiscitis is a rare medical condition, so it is very difficult and the condition is often at times misdiagnosed as back pain can be caused due to numerous medical conditions. Some of the tests which the primary physician may conduct in order to diagnose Spondylodiscitis are:

- PET/CT scan
- MRI
- Tissue biopsy
- PCR (Polymerase Chain Reaction) test

Treatment

- Conservative treatment – It may include the extensive course of antibiotics to get rid of the infection causing the disease
- Immobilization of the vertebral bodies - To allow them to get back to their normal shape
- Physical therapy
- Use of NSAIDs – In case of pain
- Surgery – To correct the defect, especially the kyphotic deformity, if conservative treatment fails

3.1.6 Pott's disease

Pott's disease, also known as tuberculosis spondylitis, is an uncommon infectious disease of the spine which is typically caused by an extra spinal infection. It is one of the oldest demonstrated diseases of humankind, having been documented in spinal remains from the Iron Age in Europe and in ancient mummies from Egypt and the Pacific coast of South America. In 1779, "Percivall Pott", (1714–1788), a British surgeon, for whom the disease is named, presented the classic description of spinal tuberculosis.

Pott's disease is a combination of osteomyelitis and arthritis which usually involves more than one vertebra. The lower thoracic and upper lumbar vertebrae are the areas of the spine most often affected. It is most commonly localized in the thoracic portion of the spine. A possible effect of this disease is vertebral collapse and when this occurs anteriorly, anterior wedging results, leading to kyphotic deformity of the spine.

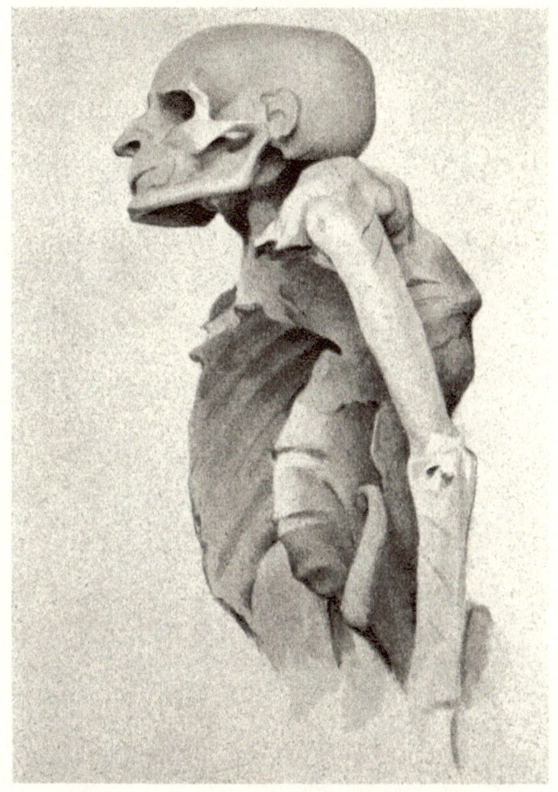

Figure 3.4: Pott's disease in a mummy

Cause

Pott's disease results from haematogenous spread of tuberculosis from other sites, often pulmonary. The infection then spreads from two adjacent vertebrae into the adjoining intervertebral disc space. If only one vertebra is affected, the disc is normal, but if two are involved, the disc, which is avascular, cannot receive nutrients and collapses. The disc tissue dies and is broken down by caseation, leading to vertebral narrowing and eventually to vertebral collapse and spinal damage.

Signs and symptoms

- Spinal Involvement - Lower thoracic vertebrae are the most common area of involvement (40-50%), followed by the Lumbar spine (35-45%) and approximately 10% of Pott's disease cases involve the cervical spine.

- Neurological Signs-Neurologic abnormalities occur in 50% of cases and can include spinal cord compression with the following:

1. Paraplegia
2. Paresis
3. Impaired sensation
4. Nerve root pain
5. Cauda equina syndrome

- Back pain- Back pain is the earliest and most common symptom

- Fever

- Night sweating

- Anorexia

- Spinal mass sometimes associated with numbness, paresthesia, or muscle weakness of the legs

- Difficulty standing

- Spinal Deformities- Almost all patients with Pott's disease have some degree of spine deformity with thoracic kyphosis being the most common

Differential diagnosis

- Pyogenic osteitis of the spine

- Spinal tumors

Musculo-skeletal	Neuro-logical	Cardio-vascular	Integumentary	Uro-genital	Constitutional Symptoms
Vertebral Fractures	Paresthesia	Spinal Artery Infarction	Pressure Ulcers (Secondary)	Bowel Dys-function	Fever
Vertebral Collapse	Paralysis	Avascularity of Intervertebral Discs	Sinus (Secondary to Abscess Rupture)	Bladder Dys-function	Night Sweats
Pinal Ligament Destruction	Paresis	Thrombosis	Cutaneous Fungal Infections		Malaise
Intervertebral Disc Destruction	Abnormal Muscle Tone				Weight Loss
Paravertebral Abscess	Abnormal Reflexes				
Osteopenia/ Osteoporosis	Cauda Equina Syndrome				
Bone Sequestrations	Myelo-malacia				
Dislocated Vertebrae	Gliosis				
Kyphotic Deformity	Syringo-myelia				
Muscle Atrophy					
Torticollis					

Figure 3.5: Systemic Signs and Symptoms of Pott's disease

Diagnosis

Diagnosis can be done by doing following tests-

- CBC - leukocytosis
- ESR – Elevated (around 100 mm/h)

- Tuberculin skin test - In 84–95% of patients with Pott disease, results are positive, who are not infected with HIV.
- X-Ray of the spine
- Bone scan
- CT of the spine
- Bone biopsy
- MRI

Treatment

- Anti-Tubercular drugs
- Analgesics
- Immobilization of the spine region by using braces and collars
- Thoracic spinal fusion
- Physical therapy & Exercises
- Surgery - To drain spinal abscesses to stabilize the spine

3.2 Non- inflammatory Spondylopathy

Spondylopathies which are degenerative but not inflammatory are called non-inflammatory spondylopathies.

3.2.1 Spondylosis

Spondylosis is a form of osteoarthritis that develops in the spine. It is degenerative, not inflammatory, as it is characterized by degradation in the cartilage within the spinal joints, which may lead to bones rubbing against one another. Additionally, it can lead to compression of nerve roots of the spinal cord. Spondylosis can occur in any part of the spine, including in the cervical (neck) region of the spine.

Causes

Spondylosis can affect a person at any age; however, older people are more susceptible, as it is an aging disorder. With age, there is wear and tear in the bones and ligaments of the spine which leads to bone spurs (osteoarthritis), degeneration of inter-vertebral discs, disc herniation and bulging of discs.

Symptoms

Many people with spondylosis in X-ray do not have any symptoms. In fact, lumbar spondylosis is present in 27%-37% of people without any symptoms. Following are the symptoms which can be felt by ailing person -

- Pain felt locally in the affected area or at a distance away
- Stiffness

- weakness,
- gait dysfunction, loss of balance,
- Loss of bowel and/or bladder control.
- The patient may experience a phenomenon of shocks (paresthesia) in hands and legs because of nerve compression and lack of blood flow

Diagnosis

- **Cervical Compression Test**is performed by laterally flexing the patient's head and placing downward pressure on it. A positive sign is neck or shoulder pain on the ipsilateral side, that is, the side to which the head is laterally flexed. This is somewhat predictive of cervical spondylosis.
- **Lhermitte sign:**feeling of electrical shock with patient neck flexion.
- Reduced range of motion of the neck, the most frequent objective finding on physical examination.
- X-rays can show bone spurs on vertebral bodies in the spine, thickening of facet joints and narrowing of the inter-vertebral disc spaces.

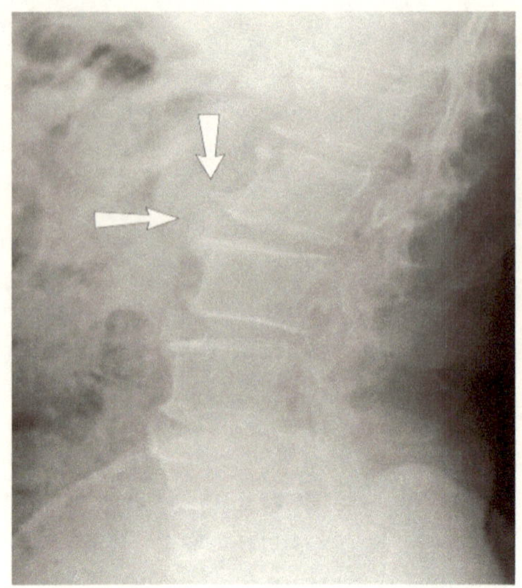

Figure 3.6: Lumbar spine spondylosis

- MRI and CT scans are helpful for pain diagnosis but generally are not definitive and must be considered together with physical examinations and history.

Treatment

Treatment is usually conservative in nature.

- Lifestyle modifications (like posture correction)
- Non-steroidal anti-inflammatory drugs (NSAIDs)
- Physical Therapy and chiropractic care
- Surgery in later stage

Complications

A major problem related to this disease is vertebrobasilar insufficiency. This is a result of the vertebral artery becoming occluded as it passes up in the transverse foramen. The spinal joints become stiff in cervical spondylosis. Thus the chondrocytes which maintain the disc become deprived of nutrition and die. The weakened disc bulges and grows out as a result of incoming osteophytes.

3.2.2 Spondylolysis

Spondylolysis is a specific defect in the connection between vertebrae, the bones that make up the spinal column. It is a result of a defect or stress fracture in the pars inter-articularis of the vertebral arch that can weaken the bones so much that one slips out of place, a condition called spondylolisthesis. The great majority of cases occur in the lowest of the lumbar vertebrae (L5), but it may also occur in the other part of spine including thoracic and cervical vertebrae.
The word spondylolysis comes from the Greek words ‘spondylos’, which means spine or vertebra, and ‘lysis’, which means a break or loosening. Spondylolysis is a very common cause of low back pain.

Causes

Spondylolysis is generally more common in males compared to females. It results from a weakness in a section of the vertebra called the pars interarticularis, the thin piece of bone that connects the upper and lower

segments of the facet joints. Facet joints link the vertebrae directly above and below to form a working unit that permits movement of the spine.
The exact cause of the weakness of the pars interarticularis is unknown. Heredity or trauma to the lower back can be the reason.

Symptoms of Spondylolysis

- Unilateral low back pain
- Pain may radiate to buttock or thigh
- Pain that worsens after strenuous activity
- Pain eased by rest.
- In 80% cases, the patient will often have an exaggerated back arch and tight hamstrings

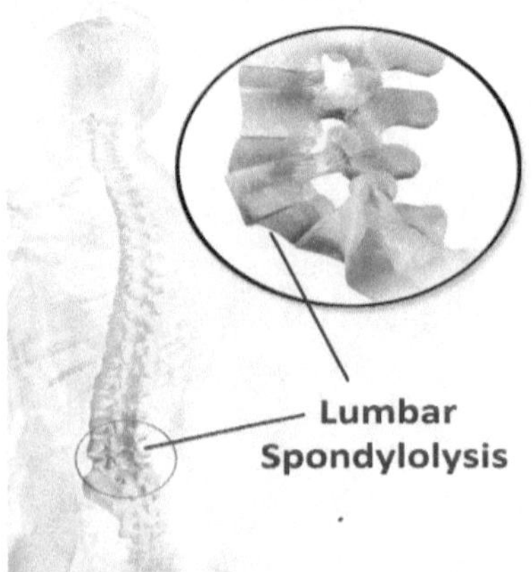

Figure 3.7: Lumbar spondylolysis

Diagnosis

- X-ray
- MRI
- Bone Scintigraphy (Bone Scan)
- Computed Tomography (CT scan)
- **One-legged hyperextension test** -It involves having the patient stand upon one leg and then leans backwards. The test should produce pain on the same side of the spine as the leg that you are standing on. If it produces pain this indicates spondylolysis on that side. The test is then performed on the other side assessing for pain again. The test can be positive on one side, both sides and neither.

Treatment

- Bracing - To immobilize the spine for a short period to allow the pars defect to heal
- Medication - Pain killers and anti-inflammatory medication
- Stretching - Starting with gentle hamstring stretching and progressing with additional stretches over time
- Exercise that is controlled and builds gradually over time

- Surgery - In rare conditions, surgery may be required to provide internal fixation and stability to the area. Usually, two procedures are performed as part of the sàme surgery:

    1. **De-compressive laminectomy** –It help to reduces irritation and inflammation in the area (but increases spinal instability)

    2. **Posterior Lumbar Spinal Fusion** -A spinal fusion to provide stabilization of the affected area

3.2.3 Spondylolisthesis

The term Spondylolisthesis is originally derived from two Greek words, "spondylos" for spine and "(o)listhesis" for forward gliding. Therefore, it means the "forward slipping of the spine". In 1854, Herman Friedrich Kilian (1800-1863) coined the term "Spondylolisthesis". Spondylolisthesis is a condition of the spine whereby one of the vertebra slips forward or backward compared to the next vertebra.

- **Anterolisthesis:** -Forward slippage of an upper vertebra on a lower vertebra.

- **Retrolisthesis:** -Backward slippage of an upper vertebra on a lower vertebra.

Spondylolisthesis can lead to a deformity of the spine as well as a narrowing of the spinal canal (central spinal stenosis) or compression of the exiting nerve roots (foraminal stenosis).

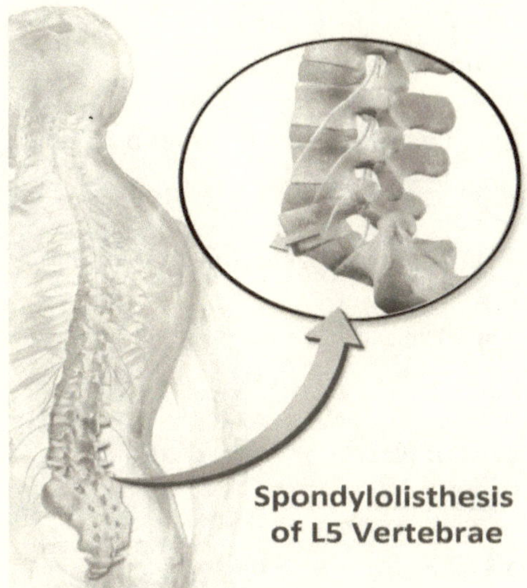

Figure 3.8: Spondylolisthesis

Causes

- Trauma or Injury
- Degenerative changes in Spine
- Tumor
- A joint damaged by an infection or arthritis
- Birth Defects (congenital)

Symptoms of spondylolisthesis

- Pain in back or buttock
- Difficulty walking
- Pain that runs from the lower back down one or both legs.
- Numbness or weakness in one or both legs.
- Leg, back, or buttock pain that gets worse when you bend over or twist.
- Loss of bladder or bowel control, in rare cases.

Diagnosis

- X-ray
- MRI
- Computed Tomography (CT scan)

Treatment

- Avoid any physical activity that may have led to vertebrae damage
- Medication - Pain killers and NSAID
- Physical therapy - To build up stomach and back muscles (core strengthening)

- Surgery - Degenerative spondylolisthesis with spinal stenosis is one of the most common indications for spine surgery among older adults

3.2.4 Spinal stenosis

It is the narrowing of spaces in the spine (backbone) which causes pressure on the spinal cord and nerves. About 75% of cases of spinal stenosis occur in the low back (lumbar spine). In most cases, the narrowing of the spine associated with stenosis compresses the nerve root, which can cause pain along the back of the leg.

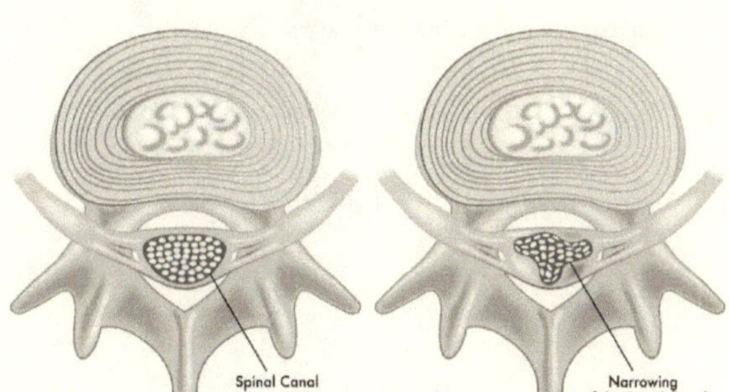

Figure 3.9: Spinal Stenosis

Types

- **Lumbar Stenosis:** In lumbar stenosis, the spinal nerve roots in the lower back are compressed, or choked, and this can produce symptoms of sciatica -- tingling, weakness or numbness that radiates from the low back and into the buttocks and legs - especially with activity.

- **Cervical Stenosis:**Cervical stenosis can be far more dangerous by compressing the spinal cord. Spinal cord stenosis may lead to serious symptoms, including major body weakness or even paralysis. Such severe spinal stenosis symptoms are virtually impossible in the lumbar spine, because the spinal cord is not present in the lumbar spine.

Causes

- Some possible causes are:
- Aging
- Ankylosing spondylitis
- Heredity
- Congenital spinal stenosis
- Osteoarthritis
- Rheumatoid arthritis
- Instability of the spine, or spondylolisthesis
- Tumors of the spine
- Trauma/ Injuries of spine

Symptoms

- Low back pain as well as pain in the legs
- Frequent falling due to lack of balance, clumsiness
- Pain and difficulty when walking
- Numbness, tingling, hot or cold feelings in the legs

Diagnosis

- X-ray
- CT scan
- MRI
- Electro myelogram – To check the nerve health

Treatment

- Changes in posture - Flexing the spine by leaning forward while walking relieves symptoms. These positions enlarge the space available to the nerves and may make it easier for people with stenosis to walk longer distances.
- Medications - Non-steroidal anti-inflammatory medications (NSAIDS) may help relieve symptoms.
- Rest

- Surgery - If other treatments do not ease the pain, surgery may be recommended to relieve the pressure on affected nerves.

3.2.5 Facet syndrome

Facet syndrome is an articular disorder of facet joints and their innervations. It results in stemming of pain which can be local or radiating. The facet joints become inflamed and may cause pain, soreness and stiffness. 55% of facet syndrome cases occur in cervical vertebrae, and 31% in lumbar. Facet syndrome can progress to spinal osteoarthritis, which is also known as spondylosis.

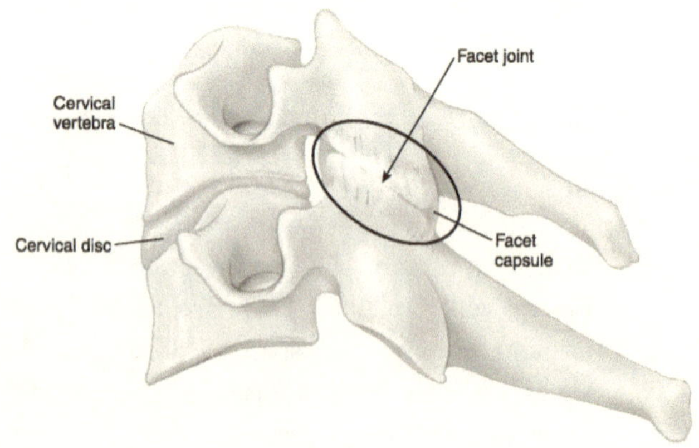

Figure 3.10: Facet Joint syndrome

Causes

- Osteoarthritis

- Facet Degeneration
- Facet Joint Injury
- Synovial Cysts
- Obesity
- Sedentary life style

Symptoms

Symptoms are depending entirely on the location of the degenerated spinal joint, severity of injury and pressure on the surrounding structures.

- Pain in the lower back (one side or both side) that can radiate into the buttocks and legs.
- Pain is worsened by stress on the facet joints and relieved by bending forward (spinal flexion).
- Neck pain that radiates into the shoulders or head.
- Pain in head at the base of the skull, aching behind the eyes.
- The sound of bone rubbing on bone when you move.

Diagnosis

- X-ray of the Spine

- MRI scan
- CT scan of Spine
- A diagnostic block into the facet joint (facet joint injection)

Treatment

- Medications - Anti-inflammatory medications for pain & inflammation
- Physical Therapy
- Facet Joint Injections - A heat injection procedure called radiofrequency ablation is used to treat facet joint syndrome. Its goal is to block the nerves that send pain from the facet joints

CHAPTER 4

INTER-VERTEBRAL DISC DISORDER

4.1 Schmorl's nodes

Schmorl's nodes, classically known as intervertebral disc herniations, are protrusions of the cartilage (nucleus pulposus) of the inter-vertebral disc through the vertebral body endplate and into the adjacent vertebra. The protrusions may contact the marrow of the vertebra, leading to inflammation.
Schmorl's node is named after German pathologist Christian Georg Schmorl (1861–1932), who first described them in 1927.

Pathology

It is believed that Schmorl nodes develop following back trauma, although this is incompletely understood. A more recent study suggests nucleus pulposus pressure on the weakest part of the end plate or vertebral development process during early life as possible explanation.

Diagnosis

- X-ray of the Spine

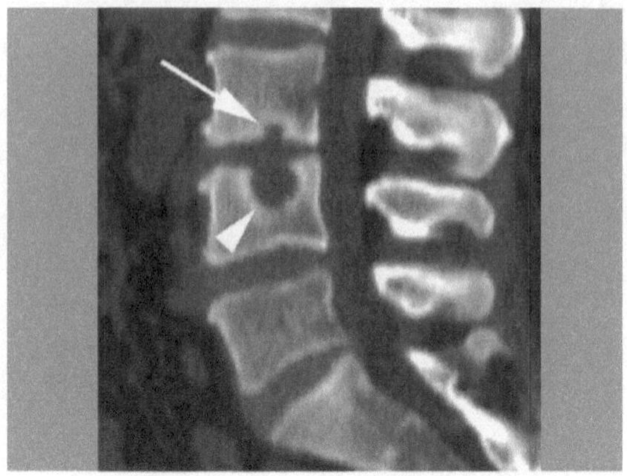

Figure 4.1: Schmorl's nodes

- MRI scan
- Computed Tomography (CT scan) of Spine

Treatment

Schmorl's nodules typically do not require extensive treatment.
However, pain is usually relieved through rest.

4.2 Degenerative disc disease

Degenerative disc disease is an age-related condition which is not really a disease but a term used to describe the normal changes in the spinal discs as we age. Degenerative disc disease can take place throughout the spine, but it most often occurs in the discs in the lower back (lumbar region) and the neck (cervical region).

Causes

As described above, it is a result of age-related changes in the spine. These changes include:

- **Loss of fluid in the discs -**This reduces the ability of the discs to act as shock absorbers and makes them less flexible. Loss of fluid also makes the disc thinner and narrows the distance between two vertebrae.

- **Wear and tear in the outer layer of the disc -** The jellylike material inside the disc (nucleus) may be forced out through the tears or cracks in the capsule, which causes the disc to bulge, break open (rupture), or break into fragments.

Symptoms

- Pain in the neck that may radiate to the arms and hands

- Chronic low backache which sometimes radiates to the hips

- Functional problems such as tingling or numbness in the legs or buttocks,

- Difficulty in walking

- Numbness and tingling in the extremities

- Weakness in the leg muscles or foot drop may be a sign that there is damage to the nerve root

Diagnosis

- A diagnosis is based on a physical examination and medical history
- X-ray
- An MRI to see the damage to discs, but it alone cannot confirm degenerative disc disease

Treatment

- Medications - Anti-inflammatory medications such as NSAID and epidural steroid injections
- Physical Therapy
- Heat and cold therapy
- Spinal mobilization
- Surgery- Artificial disc replacement, spinal fusion

4.3 Spinal disc herniation

Spinal disc herniation is a medical condition affecting the spine in which a tear in the outer, fibrous ring of an inter-vertebral disc allows the soft, central portion to bulge out beyond the damaged outer rings. Some time, it is also referred as a "slipped disc".

Pathology

A disk begins to herniate when its jelly-like nucleus pushes against its outer ring due to wear and tear or a sudden injury. This pressure against the outer ring may cause lower back pain. The most common location for a herniated disc to occur is in the disc at the level between the fourth and fifth lumber vertebrae in the low back.

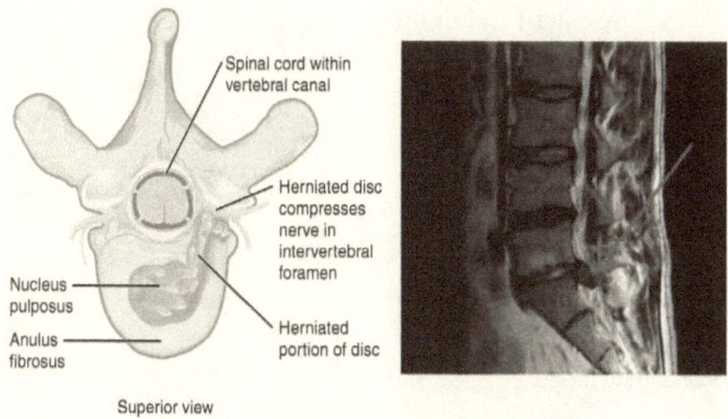

Figure 4.2: Spinal disc herniation

In many cases, a herniated disk is related to the natural aging of the spine.

Symptoms

- Back pain
- Leg and foot pain (sciatica)
- Numbness or a tingling sensation in the leg and foot
- Weakness in the leg and foot
- Loss of bladder or bowel control (extremely rare). This may indicate a more serious problem

called 'cauda equina' syndrome. This condition is caused due to compression of the spinal nerve roots. It requires immediate medical attention.

Diagnosis

- X-ray of the Spine
- MRI scan
- Computed Tomography (CT Scan) of Spine
- Myelogram - Sometimes a myelogram is necessary

Treatment

- Rest - Bed rest for one or two days can reduce the severe back pain. Sudden movements like bending forward and lifting may cause severe pain, so should be avoided.
- Medications - Anti-inflammatory medications such as NSAID and Epidural steroid injection to reduce local inflammation.
- Physical Therapy - It will help to strengthen the lower back and abdominal muscles.
- Surgery - Some patients may require surgery in severe cases.

CHAPTER 5

PAINS

5.1 Sciatica

The word "Sciatica" is derived from a Greek word "ishion" standing for hip, buttocks, sacrum, loin and also upper limb. Since the time of Hippocrates of Cos (460-370 B.C), this term has related to the pain syndrome of the lower back and the upper parts of the lower limbs. Sciatica is a name given to pain caused by pressure placed on the sciatic nerve, resulting from herniation of one or more lumbar inters- vertebral discs. Sciatic neuralgia is defined as 'pain in the distribution of the sciatic nerve due to pathology of the nerve itself'.

Sciatica Nerve

The sciatic nerve runs from the lower back, down through the hips and buttocks and along the back of the leg into the foot. It actually originates from the L4 through S3 spinal nerves. It innervates the deep muscles of the buttocks and hips. It also serves the muscles of the hamstring group, the lower leg, and some of the muscles of the foot.

Patho-physiology of sciatica

The exact patho-physiologic mechanisms behind sciatica are incompletely known; however, compression of spinal nerve roots is known to be correlated to both pain and neural dysfunction in a segmental distribution of that specific nerve root. Compression per se may impair the transport of nutrients to the nerve tissue in such a way that affects the nerve root function. There also might be a local effect on nerve roots or root sleeves by substances leaking from the degenerated inter-vertebral discs.

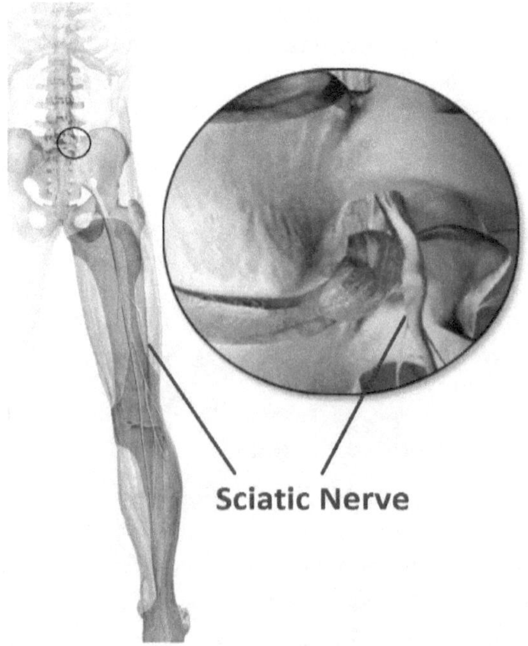

Figure 5.1: Sciatica

Causes

- Spinal disc herniation
- Spinal stenosis
- Piriformis syndrome
- Degenerative disc disease
- Sacroiliac joint dysfunction
- Pregnancy
- Spinal Tumors

Symptoms

- Pain in the rear or leg that is worse when sitting
- Burning or tingling down the leg
- Weakness, numbness, or difficulty moving the leg or foot
- A constant pain on one side of the rear
- A shooting pain that makes it difficult to stand up

Diagnosis

Sciatica is typically diagnosed by physical examination called straight-leg-raising test in which the leg is raised to a 45 degrees angle, and the history of the symptoms.

Investigation

- X-rays - To find out a bone spur that may be pressing a nerve
- CT scan
- MRI
- Electromyography (EMG) - To find out any nerve compression caused by herniated disks or narrowing of spinal canal (spinal stenosis)

Treatment

If bed rest and other self-care measures do not improve the condition, following treatment is required:

- Medication - Pain reliever, anti-inflammatories, muscle relaxants and anti-depressant for reducing the inflammation.
- Physical therapy
- Corticosteroids - These steroids injections help reduce pain by suppressing inflammation around the irritated nerve.
- Surgery - In an advance case, surgery can help to remove the bone spur or the portion of the herniated disk that's pressing on the pinched nerve.

5.2 Radiculopathy

Radiculopathy, also known as 'pinched nerve', refers to a set of conditions in which one or more nerves are affected and do not work properly due to the compression of that nerve in the spine that can cause pain, numbness, tingling or weakness along the course of the nerve.

Types

Radiculopathy can occur in any part of the spine. Radiculopathy can have different symptoms and different names depending on where in the spine it occurs.

- **Lumbar radiculopathy** -When radiculopathy occurs in the lower back, it is known as lumbar radiculopathy. Radiculopathy is most common in the lower back and the common cause of sciatica.

- **Cervical radiculopathy** -When there is a compression of nerve root in the neck region, then it is called cervical radiculopathy.

- **Thoracic radiculopathy** -It is least common location for radiculopathy and refers to a compressed nerve root in the thoracic area of the spine.

In a radiculopathy, the problem occurs at or near the root of the nerve, shortly after its exit from the spinal cord. However, the pain or other symptoms often radiate to the other part of the body served by that nerve.

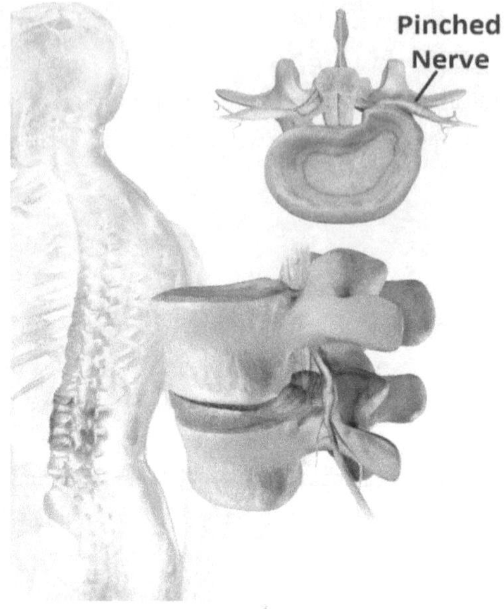

Figure 5.2: Radiculopathy

Causes

Radiculopathy is a mechanical compression of a nerve root usually at the exit foramen or lateral recess. It may due to -

- Degenerative disc disease
- Osteoarthritis
- Facet joint degeneration

- Ligamentous hypertrophy
- Spondylolisthesis
- Nerve root injuries

More rare causes of radiculopathy may include -

- Radiation
- Diabetes mellitus
- Neoplastic disease
- Meningeal-based disease process
- Herpes

Symptoms

When a nerve root is compressed, it becomes inflamed and can produce some symptoms that may include:

- Sharp pain in the back, arms, legs or shoulders that may worsen with slightest movement in body like sneezing and coughing
- Weakness or loss of reflexes in the arms or legs
- Numbness of the skin with "pins and needles" like sensations (paresthesia) in the arms or legs

The symptoms depend on the location of the spine where the nerve root is pinched.

Diagnosis

The diagnosis of radiculopathy begins with a medical history and physical examination by the physician. It includes type and location of symptoms, how long they have been present, what makes them better and worse, and what other medical problems present.

Investigation

- X-rays
- CT scan
- MRI
- Electromyogram (EMG) – To find out any damage to the nerve

Treatment

Treatment will depend on the location and the cause of the condition as well as many other factors.

- Medications - NSAID, muscle relaxants or steroid injections to reduce inflammation and relieve pain

- Exercises - Weight loss exercises to reduce pressure on the affected area
- Physical therapy - To strengthen the muscles and prevent further damage
- Surgery - To reduce the pressure on nerve root

CHAPTER 6

DIAGNOSTIC TEST USED FOR SPINAL DISORDERS

6.1 History

To design a treatment plan for the patient, a complete history of the present complaint is necessary. Suppose, if patient is having pain, it may be because of several possible internal causes. After taking the complete history, physician will get a better idea of the possible cause, and can recommend the further investigations and diagnostic tests.
Some typical questions that can be asked:

- Where is the sight of pain? What is the intensity?
- When did the pain begin?
- Is there any injury that could be related to the pain?
- Does the pain radiate to other parts of the body?

- What are the factors which make the pain feel better or worse?

- Is there a history of osteoporosis in your family?

6.2 Physical examination

After taking the complete history, physical examination allows the doctor to rule out possible causes of pain and try to determine the source of problem. The part of the body that will be examined depend upon the site where patient is experiencing the pain like nape of neck, lower back, arms, legs, etc. A typical physical examination includes following things:

- **Movement of neck and spine** -Is there any pain on twisting, bending, or moving? If so, where? Is there any loss of some flexibility?

- **Weakness** -Testing of strength of muscles by pushing or lifting the arm, hand, or leg when light resistance is put against them.

- **Pain** -Checking of the tenderness of certain part of the body.

- **Sensory Changes** -Asking about any certain sensations in specific areas?

- **Reflex changes** -Testing of tendon reflexes, such as under the kneecap and under the Achilles tendon on the ankle.

- **Motor skills** -Ask to do a toe or heel walk.

6.3 Laboratory tests

Further pathological tests may be required to determine the presence of serious problems such as an infection, arthritis, cancer, or an aortic aneurysm. A sample of blood or joint fluid helps to rule out any metabolic abnormalities, such as:

- A blood sample showing high blood levels of rheumatoid factor (RA) or having antibody called anti-cyclic citrullinated peptide antibody (anti-CCP) may suggest rheumatoid arthritis.

- High levels of antinuclear antibodies (ANAs), could suggest lupus or another inflammatory disease.

- For people with arthritis of the spine, a finding of a specific genetic marker in blood called HLA-B27 can help in diagnosis of a spondylarthropathy, such as ankylosing spondylitis or reactive arthritis.

- Tests of fluid drawn from the joint with a needle may reveal crystals of uric acid, confirming a diagnosis of gout, or a bacterium, suggesting that joint inflammation is caused by an infection.

6.4 X-rays

An x-ray (radiograph) is a noninvasive medical test that helps physicians to diagnose and treat medical conditions. Imaging with x-rays involves exposing a part of the body to a small dose of ionizing radiation to produce pictures of the inside of the body. X-rays are the oldest and most frequently used form of medical imaging.

X-rays are performed to diagnose any bone injuries or out growth by using electromagnetic beams to get the images of tissues, bones, and organs. Spinal X-rays are done to check the curve of your spine or for spinal defects.

An X-ray is used:

- To diagnose any fracture in bones or to find out any joint dislocation.
- To guide orthopedic surgeon, to perform spine repair/fusion, joint replacement and fracture reductions.
- To look for injury, infection, arthritis, abnormal bone growths and bony changes seen in metabolic conditions.
- To helps to detect and diagnose bone cancer.

6.5 Myelogram (Myelography)

It is a diagnostic imaging procedure which combines the use of an injected contrast substance with X-rays or computed tomography (CT) to evaluate abnormalities of the spinal canal, the spinal cord, nerve roots, and other tissues. A contrast dye and X-rays or computed tomography (CT) is used in this test to look for problems

in the spinal canal, spinal cord, nerve roots, and other tissues.
It is particularly useful for assessing the spine following surgery and for assessing disc abnormalities in patients who cannot undergo MRI.

6.6 Magnetic Resonance Imaging (MRI)

It is a diagnostic imaging procedure that combines the use of a large magnet, radio frequencies, and a computer to produce detailed images of soft tissues within the body. Bones do not obscure the images. Currently, MRI is the most sensitive imaging test available for the spine.
MRI helps to detect following conditions:

- Alignments and anatomy of spine.
- Any birth defects in spine or spinal cord.
- Any injury to the bone, disc, ligament or spinal cord.
- Compression or inflammation of spinal cord and nerves.
- Any infection of the vertebrae, discs, spinal cord and surrounding muscles.
- Any overgrowth/tumors in the vertebrae, spinal cord, nerves or surrounding soft tissues.

- Other possible causes of back pain such as compression fracture, and bone swelling.

MRI of spine is also used to help any plan procedures such as decompression of a pinched nerve, spinal fusion, or steroid injections. The steroid injections relieve pain and are usually given under the guidance of x-rays and MRI.

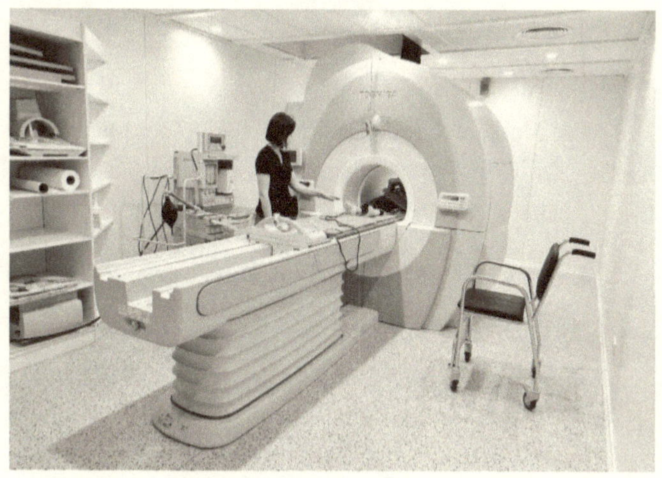

Figure 6.1: MRI Machine

6.7 Computed Tomography (CT or CAT scan)

It is a diagnostic imaging procedure that combines the use of X-rays and computer technology to produce many different views (slices) of the same body part. The images provide detailed views of bones and soft tissues. CT scanning is fast, painless, noninvasive and accurate procedure. In emergency cases, it can reveal internal injuries and bleeding quickly enough to help save lives. CT scanning of the spine is also performed to:

- Assess spine fractures due to injury.
- Evaluate the spine before and after surgery.
- Help diagnose spinal pain. One of the most common causes of spinal pain that may be diagnosed by CT is a herniated intervertebral disk.
- Measure bone density in the spine and predict whether vertebral fractures are likely to occur in patients who are at risk of osteoporosis.
- Assess for congenital anomalies of the spine or scoliosis.
- Detect various types of tumors in the vertebral column.
- Guide diagnostic procedures such as the biopsy of a suspicious area to detect cancer, or the removal of fluid from a localized infection (abscess).

In patients with narrowing (stenosis) of the spine canal, vertebral fracture, infection or degenerative disease such as arthritis, CT of the spine may provide important information when performed alone or in addition to magnetic resonance imaging (MRI).

6.8 Nerve Conduction Velocity (NCV)

Studies can detect problems with nerves, and are often used along with EMG to differentiate a nerve disorder from a muscle disorder. It measures how fast an electrical impulse moves through the nerve. NCV can identify nerve damage.

An NCV test can be used to diagnose a number of muscular and neuromuscular disorders, including:

- Guillain-Barre syndrome
- Carpal tunnel syndrome
- Charcot-Marie-Tooth (CMT) disease
- Herniated disk disease
- Chronic inflammatory polyneuropathy and neuropathy
- Sciatic nerve problems
- Peripheral nerve injury

6.9 Electromyography (EMG)

It is used to detect diseases stemming from problems with the muscle itself, and is often used with NCV to differentiate a muscle disorder from a nerve disorder. Neuromuscular abnormalities can be detected by this test.

6.10 Spinal Tap

A spinal tap is done by getting a sample of the cerebrospinal fluid that surrounds the spinal cord. The fluid contains proteins, sugar, and other substances that can be found in blood and usually is very clear. A spinal tap checks the pressure and content of the fluid. It helps to find out any problem of spinal card like any evidence of bleeding, an increase in white blood cells, an increase in protein level, or any sign of inflammation, infection, tumors, or a hemorrhage around the brain or spinal cord. To obtain the fluid sample, a needle will be inserted into the spinal canal in the lumbar region.

CHAPTER 7

YOGA AND ASANA FOR SPINE HEALTH

Yoga is an ancient science developed in India almost 4,000 years ago. Yoga is very effective for alleviating pain and stiffness related to Spine by making people more aware of how they move their bodies. Many people with back problems have found yoga very beneficial in:

- Relieving pain
- Increasing strength and flexibility of spine

Yoga is a natural and side-effect free remedy for Spinal disorders. A regular practice of yoga and different asana leads to a flexible body, calm mind and a positive attitude towards life.

Following are some yoga poses which can give you a pain-free life:

7.1 Surya Namaskar (Sun Salutation)

The person who has having the problems of neck pain, shoulder pain and cervical spondylitis and spondylosis should do Surya Namaskar, very carefully. If they perform it systematically, will gain strong and flexible spine and will be free from neck pain, shoulder pain and cervical spondylitis and spondylosis.

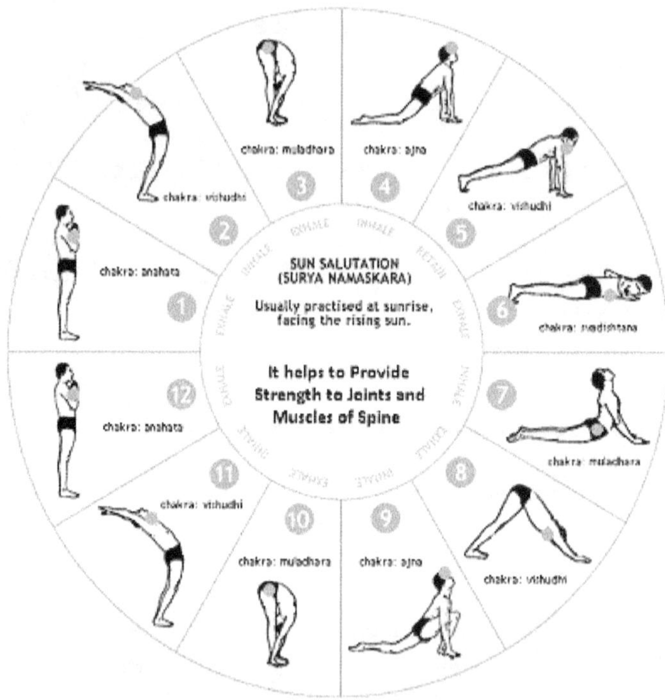

Figure 7.1: Surya Namaskar (Sun Salutation)

7.2 Matsyasana (Fish Pose)

Matsyasana provides strength and flexibility to the entire vertebral column. It is very useful asana for the muscles and tissues of cervical region and it helps in reducing the stress and strain of cervical region caused by prolong sitting in front of the computer.

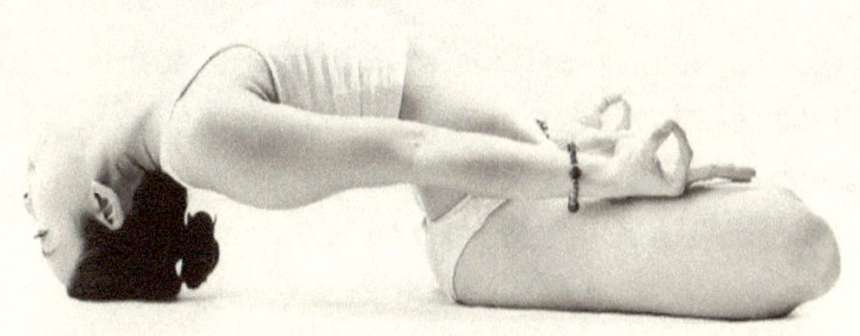

Figure 7.2: Matsyasana (Fish Pose)

7.3 Bhujangasana (Cobra Pose)

This asana decreases the stiffness of the spine. Spine is the major channel, which carries all nerve impulses from the brain to the body. Bhujangasana helps to overcome the pain & stiffness of the neck and shoulder. So, it is a useful asana for people suffering from cervical spondylitis and spondylosis.

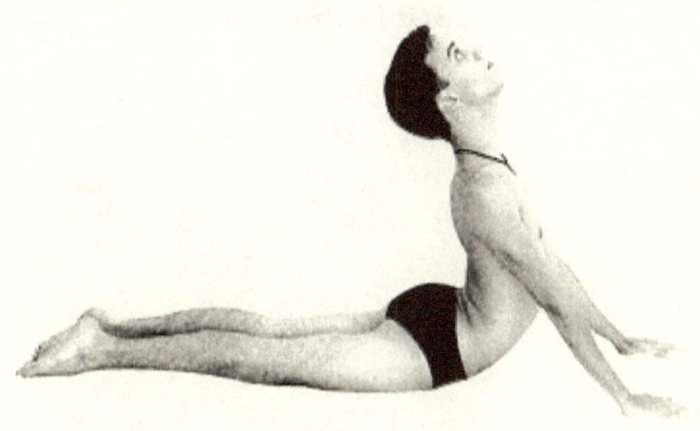

Figure 7.3: Bhujangasana (Cobra Pose)

7.4 Makarasana (Crocodile Pose)

Makarasana helps the spine to resume its normal shape and releases the nerve compression of the spine. It is effective in treating of cervical spondylitis and spondylosis, and pain of neck and shoulders.

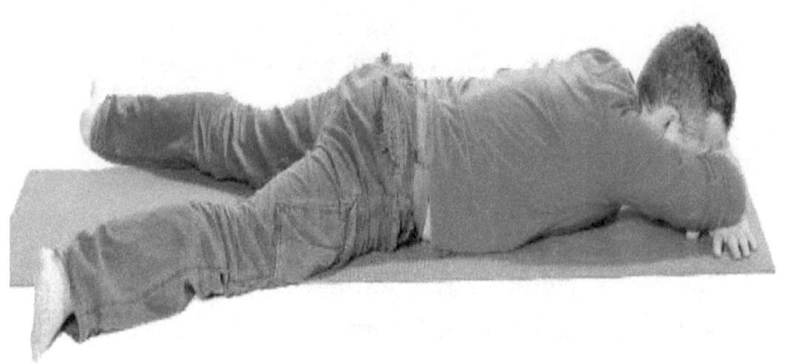

Figure 7.4: Makarasana (Crocodile Pose)

7.5 Bal-Shayanasana (Infant's Pose)

Balshayan asana is very effective asana for the patients who are suffering from lower backache or cervical spondylitis because of stress, tension and excessive workload.

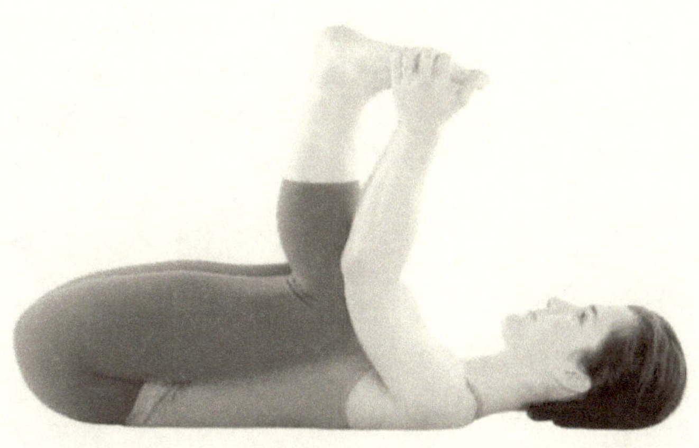

Figure 7.5: Bal-Shayanasana (Infant's Pose)

7.6 Ardha Naukasana (Half Boat Pose)

Ardha naukasana is effective for the patients of cervical & back problems. It also can help in managing chronic indigestion, constipation.

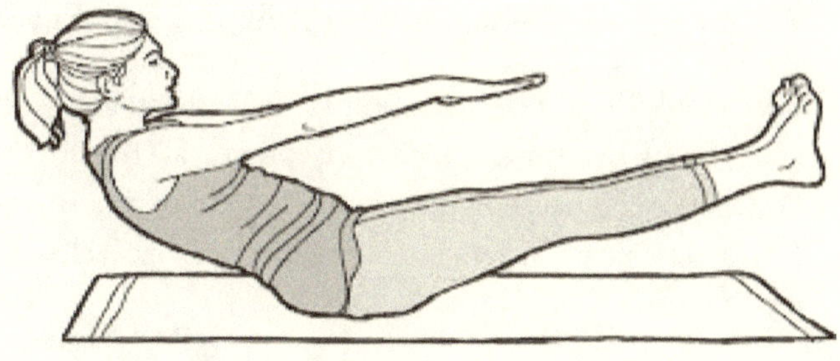

Figure 7.6: Ardha Naukasana (Half Boat Pose)

7.7 Ardha Salbhaasana (Half Locust Pose)

The gentle back extension is highly beneficial in cervical pain, lumbago and sciatica. By performing this asana regularly, patient gets a great relief from cervical spondylosis and neck pain.

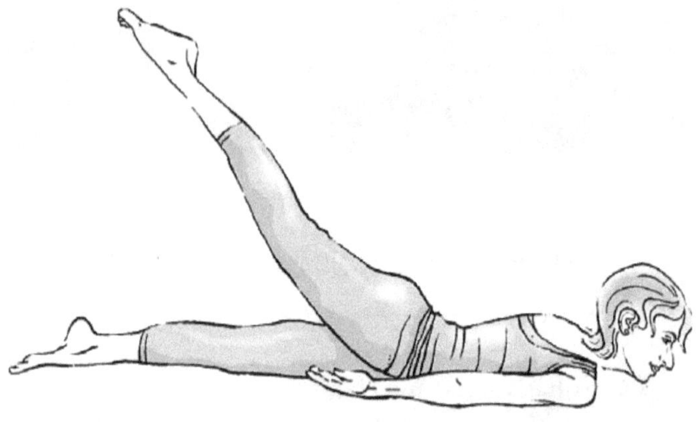

Figure 7.7: Ardha Salbhaasana (Half Locust Pose)

7.8 Shanshank-Bhujangasana (Striking Cobra Pose)

Shanshank-Bhujangasana improves flexibility and strength of the spine which can counter all the adverse effects of sedentary life. The combination of Shanshank-Bhujangasana is beneficial in treating of backache and cervical pain.

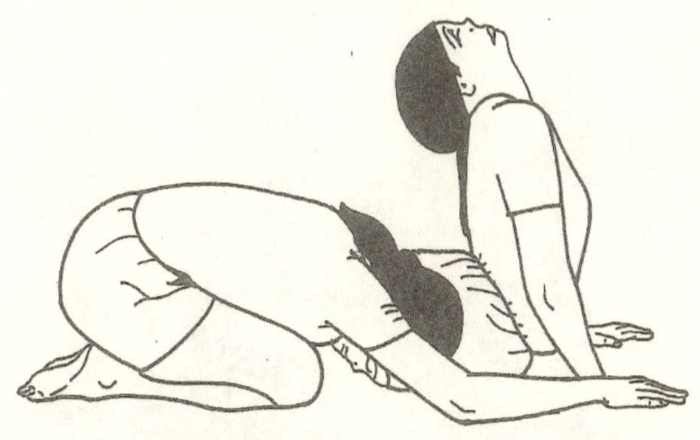

Figure 7.8: Shanshank-Bhujangasana (Striking Cobra Pose)

7.9 Kohni Chalana (Elbow Rotations)

Kohni Chalana is very useful to improve the mobility and strength of the shoulders and the neck which may prevent cervical spondylitis, frozen shoulder and bursitis.

7.10 Marjariasana (Cat Pose)

Marjariasana provides gentle massage to your spine and helps to loosen up the vertebral column. This asana is recommended to those people who are suffering from chronic neck pain and having rigid spines. Marjariasana gently stretches and stimulates the spinal nerves.

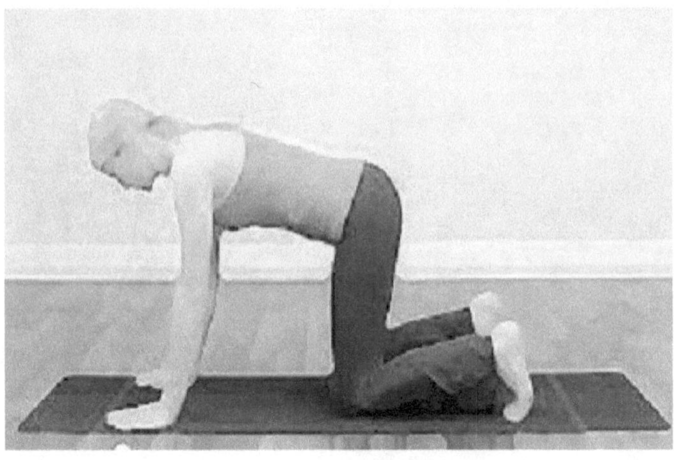

Figure 7.9: Marjariasana (Cat Pose)

Regular practicing of these yogic asana, gives strength to the spine and vertebral column. It can helps to release the nerve compression and thus alleviating pain, stiffness, vertigo and other problem related to spinal disorder.

CHAPTER 8

TIPS TO KEEPING YOUR SPINE HEALTHY

Your spine is not just a backbone but it is a part of your central nervous system. So, be kind to your spine and follow these tips for maintain the health of your spine. These are simple tips which you should keep in mind throughout the day because your spine is always on work.

8.1 Sit up straight

'Sit up straight and don't slouch', if you have to sit for long at a time. Keep your head up and your shoulders back. If you are having a habit of slouching, you are putting a lot of stress on your spine and the muscles surrounding it. Poor posture can also lead to nerve compression and limited blood flow to the surrounding area and can cause weakness of that region.

Studies say that sitting straight can help to improve digestion & breathing and person felt less depressed.

8.2 Be careful when bending and lifting

When picking up something from the floor, never bend at the waist to reach for it; instead get as close to the object as you can by kneeling down on one knee, and pick it up slowly. Even better, you should bend at the knees so that your arms are at the same height as the item. Keep your back straight. If the item is heavy, don't try to lift it yourself and get some help.

8.3 Give your spine a rest by good sleep

Sleeping well is important to your overall health. Your body needs a good night's sleep to repair itself. Sleep on your side, not your stomach. Sleeping on your stomach puts too much pressure on your spine. Whenever you lie on your back, place a pillow under your knees, which will greatly ease the pressure on your spine. If you experience any back or neck pain in bed, change positions immediately.

8.4 Stretch out and stay active

Do activities and work outs which helps to stretch your back and neck. It helps to maintain normal joint function and also reduces the risk of injury. You can make regular visits to the gym, walk, bike, swim, or play with your kids. The best exercise routine for your back and neck is one that combines stretching, strengthening, and aerobic activity. A proper exercise routine will not only strengthen your back, but also help you to lose weight or maintain a proper weight. Being overweight is not good for your spine health.

8.5 Drink water and stay hydrated

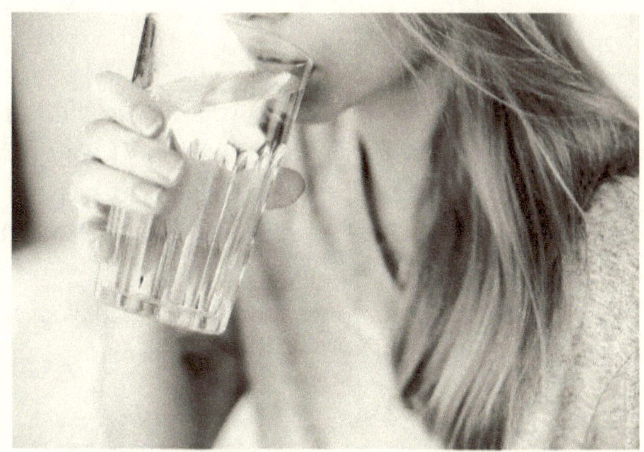

Figure 8.1: Take plenty of water

To maintain the elasticity of soft tissues and fluidity in joints, staying hydrated is very important. Intervertebral discs are vulnerable to loss of hydration and can begin to lose height. As the discs begin to shrink, you are more vulnerable to painful disc conditions such as bulging or ruptures. Drink at least eight 6-8 glasses of water daily.

8.6 Work smart and be healthy

Make sure your workspace, whether a laptop, phone, computer desk, or even your car is set up for your height and functionality. Choose a chair that provides back support. Your knees should be at 90 degrees and your feet should rest comfortably on the floor. Never cradle your phone between your ear and shoulder, to avoid this use a headset, it will help you to avoid neck pain. Take regular breaks as staying in one position for too long will cause back muscles to tighten up and become immobile which further cause stiffness and pain in back.

8.7 Listen to your body

Listen to what your body is telling you. Don't ignore the signs and symptoms of your spine problem. If your back is paining, don't medicate yourself and take help of a professional. Take a proper treatment and give rest to your spine.

Follow above tips into your daily routine and you can avoid a lot of common back and neck problems.

CHAPTER 9

DIET AND NUTRITION FOR SPINE HEALTH

Nutritious & balanced diet play a major role to keep body healthy and fit and so for Spine also. To keep a spine healthy and strong, you have to take nutritious food and should avoid food items which are harmful to your spine and body. Try to stick with a healthy diet plan that is right for you, and which can improve your spine Health.

- **Drink lot of water** -Re-hydrate yourself as fluids are important to healthy spine. Drink at least eight 6-8 glasses of water daily.
- **Avoid simple sugar** -Avoid taking sweet snacks, white flour, and starchy vegetables. Try to eat only whole grains.
- **Avoid processed foods** -This may include anything that is cooked before it is packaged. Especially try to avoid "fast food."
- **Take fresh & seasonal vegetable** -Fresh and seasonal vegetables in our daily diet promote good health of spine.

- **Include fresh fruit** -Two or three servings daily are adequate for health of spine. Avoid artificial fruit juices or fruit "drinks."

- **Add nuts and seeds** -Walnuts and pumpkins seeds provide healthy fat which is essential for spine health.

- **Chose right protein diet** -Choose fish often, and beef rarely for good spine health.

- **Healthy fat** -Olive oil can be used for cooking or added to salad to increase your healthy fat intake and thus improve health of spine.

- **Take adequate calcium in your diet** -Calcium is essential for maintaining the necessary level of bone mass to support the structures of the body.

9.1 Why we need calcium in our diet?

Calcium is needed for strong bones -Calcium is essential for maintaining the necessary level of bone mass to support the structures of the body. The body is constantly using calcium for the heart, blood, muscles and nerves. If our diet does not include enough calcium to replace what is used, the body will take calcium away from the bones, which weakens them and makes them more likely to fracture.

Calcium also prevents osteoporosis -It is especially important for children and teens to have enough calcium to aid the development of their bones and bone mass.

Later in the life, lack of sufficient calcium in the diet significantly increases the risk of developing osteoporosis (thinning of the bone).
Osteoporosis can result in fractures in the bones in the spine, which in turn can lead to chronic pain and possibly deformity. This risk of developing osteoporosis is higher in old age especially in older women.

9.2 Dietary sources of calcium

Following are the nutritional foods, which can maintain a healthy level of calcium in our body through diet alone, without using any outside supplements:

- Dairy products (e.g. yogurt, cheese and especially milk)
- Dark green leafy vegetables (e.g. spinach, broccoli and kale)
- Beans and peas (e.g. tofu, peanuts, peas, black beans)
- Some types of fish (e.g. salmon, sardines)
- Certain other foods with calcium (e.g. oranges, blackstrap molasses, almonds)

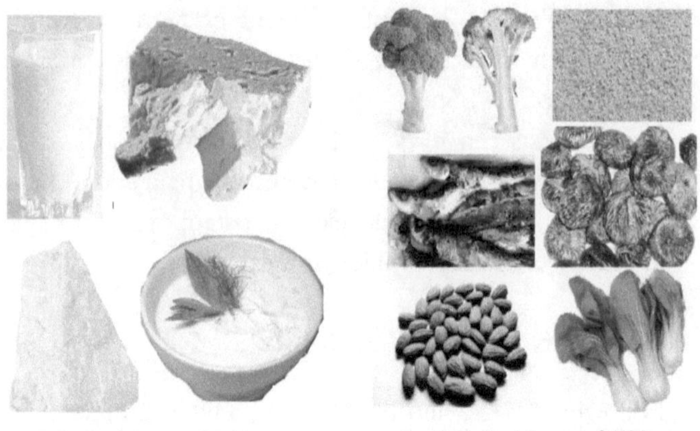

Figure 9.1: Sources of Calcium

9.3 Vegetarian sources of calcium

- Milk
- Cottage cheese
- Almonds
- Pulses (though bound to phytate)
- Seeds especially Sesame, Sunflower
- Cheddar Cheese
- Swiss Cheese
- H. Soya beans and their products like TOFU (bean curd)

9.4 Foods item which can prevent the calcium absorption and should be avoided

- Foods containing oxalic acids. E.g. spinach, lotus stem, horse gram.
- Overuse of proteins like meat, fish, poultry, eggs, etc.
- Excessive use of common salt, alcohol, coffee, tobacco, fat and soft drinks containing phosphorus.

9.5 How much calcium does your body required? *

Age	Calcium (in mg)
1-3 year old	500mg
4-8 year old	800mg
9-18 year old	1300mg
19-50 year old	1000mg
51-70 year old	1200mg
70 and older	1200mg

**** reviewed by UCSF (University of California San Francisco) Health medical specialists***

9.6 A Guide to Calcium-Rich Foods

Everybody knows that milk is a great source of calcium, but there are many different foods are available which can be added in our diet to reach daily recommended amount of calcium. Use the following list of food items especially suitable for Indian population, to get additional calcium in your diet.

CALCIUM CONTENT OF SOME COMMON FOODS	PORTION	CALCIUM*
Buttermilk	1 cup/250mL	186 mg
Fortified orange juice	1 cup/250mL	300 mg
Fortified almond, rice or soy beverage	1 cup/250mL	300 mg
Milk – whole, 2%, 1%, skim, chocolate	1 cup/250mL	300 mg
Milk, evaporated	1/2 cup/125 mL	367 mg
Milk – powder, dry	1/3 cup/75 mL	270 mg
Yogurt – plain, 1-2% M.F.	3/4 cup/175 mL	332 mg
Almonds, dry roast	1/2 cup/125 mL	186 mg

Beans – white, canned	1 cup/250 mL	191 mg
Cheese – Blue, Brick, Cheddar, Edam, Gouda, Gruyere, Swiss	1 ¼"/3 cm cube	245 mg
Cheese – Mozzarella	1 ¼"/3 cm cube	200 mg
Drinkable yogurt	4/5 cup/200 mL	191 mg
Frozen yogurt, vanilla	1 cup/250 mL	218 mg
Fruit-flavoured yogurt	3/4 cup/175 mL	200 mg
Ice cream cone, vanilla, soft serve	1	232 mg
Kefir (fermented milk drink) – plain	3/4 cup/175 mL	187 mg
Molasses, blackstrap	1 Tbsp/15 mL	180 mg
Salmon, with bones – canned	1/2 can/105 g	240 mg
Sardines, with bones	1/2 can/55 g	200 mg
Soybeans, cooked	1 cup/250 mL	170 mg
Beans – baked, with pork, canned	1 cup/250 mL	129 mg
Beans – navy, soaked, drained, cooked	1 cup/250 mL	126 mg

Collard greens – cooked	1/2 cup/125 mL	133 mg
Cottage cheese, 1 or 2%	1 cup/250 mL	150 mg
Figs, dried	10	150 mg
Instant oatmeal, calcium added	1 pouch/32 g	150 mg
Soy flour	1/2 cup/125 mL	127 mg
Tofu, regular – with calcium sulfate	3 oz/84 g	130 mg
Beans – baked, plain	1 cup/250 mL	86 mg
Beans – great northern, soaked, drained, cooked	1 cup/250 mL	120 mg
Beans – pinto, soaked, drained, cooked	1 cup/250 mL	79 mg
Beet greens – cooked	1/2 cup/125 mL	82 mg
Bok choy, Pak-choi – cooked	1/2 cup/125 mL	84 mg
Bread, white	2 slices	106 mg
Chickpeas (garbanzo beans)	1 cup/250 mL	77 mg
Chili con carne, with beans – canned	1 cup/250 mL	84 mg

Cottage cheese – 2%, 1%	1/2 cup/125 mL	75 mg
Dessert tofu	1/2 cup/100 g	75 mg
Okra – frozen, cooked	1/2 cup/125 mL	89 mg
Processed cheese slices, thin	1 slice	115 mg
Turnip greens – frozen, cooked	1/2 cup/125 mL	104 mg
Artichoke – cooked	1 medium	54 mg
Beans, snap – fresh or frozen, cooked	1/2 cup/125 mL	33 mg
Broccoli – cooked	1/2 cup/125 mL	33 mg
Chinese broccoli (gai lan) – cooked	1/2 cup/125 mL	46 mg
Dandelion greens – cooked	1/2 cup/125 mL	74 mg
Edamame (East Asian dish, baby soybeans in the pod)	1/2 cup/125 mL	52 mg
Fireweed leaves, raw	1/2 cup/125 mL	52 mg
Grapefruit, pink or red	01-Feb	27 mg
Hummus	1/2 cup/125 mL	50 mg

Kale – cooked	1/2 cup/125 mL	49 mg
Kiwifruit	1	26 mg
Mustard greens – cooked	1/2 cup/125 mL	55 mg
Orange	1 medium	50 mg
Parmesan cheese, grated	1 Tbsp/15 mL	70 mg
Rutabaga (yellow turnip) – cooked	1/2 cup/125 mL	43 mg
Seaweed (agar) – dried	1/2 cup/125 mL	35 mg
Snow peas – cooked	1/2 cup/125 mL	36 mg
Squash (acorn, butternut) – cooked	1/2 cup/125 mL	44 mg

**** The calcium content listed for most foods is estimated and can vary due to multiple factors.***

Calcium is an essential mineral for bones and overall health of the body and you may not be getting enough in your diet. Dairy products are high in calcium, but plenty of other good sources are also available out of them, most are plant-based.

Whether you are vegetarian or non-vegetarian, you have a diverse list of calcium-rich foods given in the above table. You can choose your food as per the availability and need.

CHAPTER 10

HOMOEOPATHY AND SPINAL DISORDERS

"Natural forces within us are the true healers of disease"

- HIPPOCRATES

Homoeopathy and its founder, 'Dr. Samuel Hahnemann' does not require any introduction. Homeopathy is a more than 200 years old system of medicine. Natural ingredients of Homeopathic medicines stimulate the own healing mechanisms of body so that body can heal itself. Homoeopathy strengthens the vital force of the body and provides protection from illness. Homoeopathic medicines are safe to use and when taken appropriately under the supervision of a qualified homoeopath, rarely cause any adverse effects. These medicines can be taken by patients of all ages, including infants, children, old and pregnant or breastfeeding women.

10.1 Homoeopathy

The word homoeopathy is a Greek derivation where *'homoeos'* means similar and *'pathos'* means suffering.

Homoeopathy is a system of medicine based on definite principle 'likes to be cured by likes'. In simple words, Homoeopathy treats the sufferings of a person by the administration of a drug which has been experimentally proved to possess the power of producing similar sufferings in healthy human beings i.e. on symptom similarity. Homeopathy treats each person as a unique individual with the aim of stimulating their own healing ability (immune power).

As per world health organization (WHO), Homeopathy is the 2nd largest system of medicine in the world. Worldwide, over 800 million people use homoeopathy on a regular basis and being practiced in over 80 countries.

10.2 Origin of Homoeopathy

Homoeopathy is founded by Dr. Christian Friedrich Samuel Hahnemann (10th April 1755 - 2nd July 1843), a German physician in the year 1796. For his contribution to homoeopathy, he is also known as "father of Homoeopathy".

He was a versatile genius of his era. He was an experienced orthodox physician as well a competent chemist. He did his 'Doctorate in Medicine' at the age of 24 years, from the Erlangen University. Including the German language, he was master in eight languages.

Being an orthodox physician, he was dissatisfied with the conventional medical practices of his day. Dr.

Hahnemann was disagreed to the harsh methods of treating, like blood-letting, purging and giving large doses of toxic materials such as arsenic and lead to the patients, in those days. He investigated the effects of various medicinal substances on himself and other healthy volunteers and deduced that an illness could be treated with a very small amount of a substance that, in larger quantities, could cause that illness. He termed this principle 'similia similibus curentur' or 'let likes be cured by likes'.

The principle of treating "like with like" was first backed by 'Hippocrates (460-377BC)', who also thought that symptoms specific to an individual should be taken into account before making a diagnosis. But, Dr. Hahnemann proved and practices this principle by founding Homoeopathy.

10.3 Fundamental Principles of Homoeopathy

Every science has certain fundamental principles which guide the whole system. Homoeopathy as a science of medical treatment has a philosophy of its own and its therapeutics is based on certain fundamental principles, which are also called as 'seven cardinal principles' of Homoeopathy:

- **Law of Similia** - Most similar medicine of patient's symptoms
- **Law of Simplex** - Most simple medicine for patient

- **Law of Minimum** - Minimum required medicine for patient
- **Doctrine of Drug Proving** - Homoeopathic medicine are proved on healthy human being
- **Theory of Chronic Disease** - Complex diseases comes under Psora, Sycosis and syphilis
- **Theory of Vital Force** -Body got sick due to derangement of vital force (Immune power)
- **Doctrine of Drug Dynamisation** -Power of Homoeopathic medicine has increased by Potentization

A full description of these cardinal principles of homoeopathy is very vast and explaining them here is beyond the scope of this book.

10.4 Homoeopathic management of spinal disorders

Homoeopathy sees the symptoms as the body's reaction against the illness as it attempts to overcome it, and seeks to stimulate and not suppress this reaction. Thus, it concentrates on treating the patient rather than the disease or in other words it builds up the body's immune system to fight against the disease.

Homeopathy is the only form of treatment that has demonstrated an overwhelming positive response in treating Spinal Disorders. In the event of Spinal disorders, Homoeopathic medicines not only relieve the symptoms of pain, stiffness and numbness that are commonly seen but also allow the patient to regain complete mobility and flexibility.

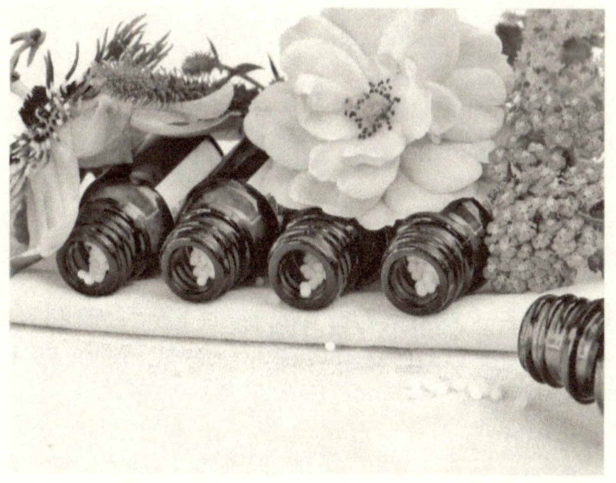

Figure 10.1: Homoeopathic medicines

Homoeopathy works on the principal of 'individualization' and 'miasm'. As per this approach, a remedy is selected which matches all the symptoms of a suffering patient and stimulates his vital force to restore balance and health. It helps to stop the further demineralization and degeneration process of the bones of the affected joint. By giving power & strength to the connecting ligaments and tendons, it strengthens the whole joint. It also helps to remove the nerve compression of spine and maintain the space between the vertebrae. Homoeopathic medicines also prevent the fusion of joints and the further spreading of disease in adjoining organs. In advance stage, where destruction of the joint has been achieved, homoeopathy can stop the further destruction and maintain the wellbeing of the patient without any harmful effects on the body.

10.5 Some Homoeopathic remedies

Following are some homoeopathic medicines which are very useful in treating the Spinal disorders-

ARNICA MONTANA

Arnica is an effective medicine for gout and chronic arthritis with a feeling of bruised soreness required this remedy.
Indications:

- Pain is worse from touch and may occur in joints that were injured in the past.
- Pain in back and limbs, as if bruised or beaten. Everything on which he lies seems too hard.
- Due to bruised pain in the pelvic region, the patient cannot walk erect.

Modalities:
Aggravation from - From least touch; motion; rest; wine and damp cold.
Amelioration from – Better by pressure, lying down, or with head low.

BRYONIA ALBA

Bryonia is very effective homeopathic remedy for stitching, tearing and aching like pain in every muscle. It is useful for the person who is having constitution of a robust, firm fiber and dark complexion, with tendency to leanness and irritability.

Indications:

- Pain and stiffness in the nape of neck.
- Stitches, stiffness and tearing pain in back which increase on slight movement.
- Joints become red, swollen, hot and painful, especially of right side.

Modalities:

Aggravation from - From warmth, hot weather, slight movement and motion, physical exertion, eating, touch and sudden change in weather.

Amelioration from - Pressure, rest, cold things and lying on painful side.

CALCAREA CARBONICA

It is the most successful remedy in several cases with rigidity & stiffness in morning, difficulty in turning with tendency to strain easily.

Indications:

- Weakness of Spine.
- Stiffness and rigidness of nape of neck.

- Backache as if sprained from over lifting which cause difficulty in rising from the bed.
- Pain between the shoulders which case difficulty in breathing.

Modalities:
Aggravation from - From physical exertion, cold in every form, water, washing, wet weather, standing and in full moon.
Amelioration from - Dry climate, lying on painful side.

CALCAREA FLUORICA

Calcarea fluorica is a powerful tissue remedy for malnutrition of bones.
Indications:

- Indicated for chronic lumbago (pain in lower back) which is aggravated on beginning to move, and ameliorated on continued motion.
- Burning pain in lower part of back.
- Overgrowth and tumors of bones.
- Chronic synovitis of knee-joint.

Modalities:
Aggravation from - From rest, changes of weather and beginning to move.
Amelioration from - From heat, warm applications and

by continued motion.

CALCAREA PHOSPHORICA

A great remedy for non-union of fractured bones when bones become weak due to lack of nutrition.

Indication:

- Rheumatic pain in the cervical region from draught of air, with stiffness and dullness of head.
- Pain and soreness in sacro-iliac symphysis, as it has been broken.
- Numbness and cold feeling in the back and extremities with pain and stiffness, which increases by every change of weather.

Modalities:

Aggravation from - From exposure to damp, cold weather, melting snow and every change of weather.

Amelioration from - By dry and warm climate, in summer.

CAUSTICUM

It is a wonderful remedy for dark-complexioned and rigid-fibered persons. Effective in treating chronic rheumatic, arthritic and paralytic affections.

Indications:

- Useful for stiffness between the shoulders with dull pain in the nape of neck.

- Useful for the tearing, drawing pains in the muscular and fibrous tissues with deformities of the joints.

- Left-sided sciatica with numbness of affected leg. There is restlessness in legs at night.

- Paralysis of single parts which cause dull & tearing pain in hands and arms.

Modalities:

Aggravation from- From dry, cold winds, in clear fine weather, cold air, from long standing and motion of carriage.

Amelioration from – From damp, wet weather, from warmth and heat of bed.

CIMICIFUGA

Cimicifuga is mostly suitable for the person who has to sit prolonged in front of the computer like data operator, steno and IT professionals and suffering from stiffness & pain in neck. This remedy has a wide action upon the cerebrospinal and muscular system.

Indication:

- Spine is very sensitive, especially upper part of spine.

- Stiffness and contraction in neck and back.

- Electric like pain in the lumbar and sacral spine which extends to hip and thigh.

- Sensitiveness to pressure on the upper and lower cervical vertebrae.

- Aching in the lumbar region with weakness of the lower extremities.

Modalities:
Aggravation from - From cold, during menses, motion and in morning.
Amelioration from – By rest, warmth and after eating.

CONIUM MACULATUM

Conium is a very effective remedy for weakness of mind and body due to sudden loss of strength in muscles.
Indications:

- There is pain between shoulders.

- Pain and stiffness in the spine due to after effects of bruises and shocks to spine.

- Coccyodynia – There is pain in the coccyx. Dull and aching pain in lumbar and sacral region.

- Fingers and toes become numb with muscular weakness.

- Vertigo, when lying down, when turning over in bed, when turning head sidewise, or by turning eyes.

Modalities:
Aggravation from - From taking cold, mental & physical exertion, before and during menses, lying down and by turning the head on bed.
Amelioration from - While fasting, in the dark, from letting limbs hang down, motion and pressure.

GUAIACUM

A great remedy for cervical spondylitis and suitable to the person with arthritis and rheumatic diathesis.
Indications:

- There is aching & stiffness in neck with soreness in shoulders. Pain extends from head to neck.
- There is contraction of limbs with stiffness and immobility. Person always wants to stretch. The limbs.
- Contractive & rheumatic pain in shoulders, arms and hand.
- Very useful for sciatica and lumbago.

Modalities:
Aggravation from- From motion, heat, cold wet weather, pressure, touch and from 6 pm to 4 am.
Amelioration from – From external pressure.

HYPERICUM

Hypericum is a great homeopathic remedy to heal the injuries of nerve pain. Excessive painfulness is a guiding symptom to select this remedy.

Indications:

- Useful for pain in nape of neck & shoulders due to cervical spondylitis.
- There is numbness & tingling in the extremities with jerking and twitching of muscles.
- Useful for unbearable pain along the nerve pathway which radiates from one area to another.
- Very useful in Coccydynia (Pain in coccyx) which radiates up spine and down limbs.

Modalities:

Aggravation from - From cold, damp weather, in a fog, in close room, by touch and least exposure.

Amelioration from - From pressure and bending head backward.

KALMIA LATIFOLIA

This remedy is most suitable for neuralgic pains that are shifting in nature. Pain shoots downwards, with numbness of the affected parts.

Indications:

- Pain in neck which shoots down to the arm and to the shoulders.

- Pain in localized regions of spine as if it would break which goes down to back.
- Pains shift rapidly, shooting outward, along the nerves. Pain in left hand along the ulnar nerve with tingling and numbness.
- Aching, bruised, stiff feeling in the neck and the arms.
- Weakness, numbness, pricking, and sense of coldness of painful parts.

Modalities:
Aggravation from- Pain is worse from stooping, looking down, from motion, open air, from becoming cold and lying on left side.
Amelioration from – By food.

KALI CARBONICUM

This is a very effective medicine for the stiffness of the neck and back. Great remedy for the back pain that originates after labor and miscarriages.
Indications:

- Weakness feeling in the Small of back. Backs and legs give out.
- Burning, Stiffness and paralytic feeling in the spine.

- Lumbago with sudden sharp pains extending up and down back and to thighs.
- Uneasiness, heaviness, and jerking in the limbs. Tearing pain in arms from shoulder to wrist.
- Pain from hip to knee. Paralysis of old people, Limbs go to sleep easily.

Modalities:
Aggravation from - Worse after coition, exertion, cold weather, draft, from soup and coffee, in morning about three o'clock, lying on left and painful side.
Amelioration from – Better in warm weather, during day and by movement.

LACHNANTHES TINCTORIA

This is a very effective remedy for torticollis and cervical spondylitis. It is especially useful in acute pain in the region of neck.

Indications:

- Stiffness and rheumatism of neck. The neck drawn over to one side, usually the right side.
- Pain in nape of the neck as if dislocated.
- Chilliness felt in between the shoulder with pain and stiffness in back.
- The pain increases by lying down and better by walking about.

Modalities:
Aggravation from - By Turning and moving the head backward, by lying down.
Amelioration from - By movement

LYCOPODIUM

This medicine is best suited to the person who are intellectually keen, but of weak muscular power. Nearly in all cases of spine problem of lycopodium, urinary or digestive problems will be found.
Indications:

- Pain in the back with burning sensation between the scapulae, as if there is a hot coal put on the spine.
- Drawing & tearing pain with numbness in the extremities which increases at rest or at night.
- Painful sciatica, mostly of right side. Person can't lie on affected side.
- Hands and feet become numbs with twitching and jerking.

Modalities:
Aggravation from - Problems become worse mainly on right side, from right to left, from above downward, 4 to 8 pm, from heat or warmth, hot air and warm applications in general (except throat and stomach problems which are better by warm food and drink).
Amelioration from - By motion, after midnight, from

warm food and drink, on getting cold, from being uncovered.

NUX VOMICA

Nux vomica is a very good homoeopathic medicine which helps to treat many of the conditions, incident to modern life. Useful in treating neck pains & backaches due to prolong sitting in offices and sedentary life style.

Indications:

- Pain in lumbar region with burning sensation in spine, which increase in early morning (Between 3 to 4 am).
- Cervico-brachial neuralgia. Must sit-up in order to turn in bed. Bruised pain below the scapulae which make sitting painful.
- There is sudden loss of power in the legs in the morning. Legs feels numb and paralyzed. Numbness in spine and extremities.

Modalities:

Aggravation from - In morning, mental exertion, after eating, touch, spices, stimulants, narcotics, dry weather and cold.

Amelioration from - In evening, from rest, strong pressure and in damp & wet weather.

PARIS QUADRIFOLIA

A good homoeopathic remedy for the treatment of cervical spondylitis.
Indication:

- There is a sensation of weight and weariness in the nape of the neck and between the shoulders.
- Neuralgic pains that begin in the left side of the chest and radiate along the left arm.
- Stiffness of the arms with clinching of fingers due to pain in the neck.
- There is a feeling of numbness in the hands and fingers due to the cervical spondylitis. Due to this numbness in fingers, everything the patient holds feel rough.

Modalities:
Aggravation from- By touch, motion, mental exertion.
Amelioration from – By rest, open air.

PHYTOLACCA DECANDRA

It is a great homoeopathic remedy having powerful effect on fibrous and osseous tissues. Aching, soreness, restlessness and prostration are general symptoms which guide to select the phytolacca decandra.
Indications:

- Syphilitic bone pains with chronic rheumatism.

- Aching pains in lumbar region. Pains extend up and down the spine into sacrum.

- Stiffness of back and neck especially right side with shooting pain in right shoulder which cause inability to raise the arm.

- Pains fly like electric shocks, shooting, lancinating, shifting rapidly.

Modalities:
Aggravation from- By motion, in night, in cold weather, Right side, in rain, getting wet and exposure to damp weather.
Amelioration from – By warmth, dry weather and at rest.

RHUS TOXICODENDRON

It is a frequently and commonly used homoeopathic remedy for lower back pain or lumbar spondylitis. It mainly affects fibrous tissue like joints, tendons, sheaths-aponeurosis producing pains and stiffness.
Indication:

- Pain between the shoulders which aggravates by swallowing anything.

- Pain and stiffness in back which increases after sitting for long, in the morning on getting up and get relief by motion or by lying on something hard.

- Rheumatic pain and stiffness of the nape of the neck with loss of power in forearm and fingers.

- Sciatica pain aggravated by cold & damp weather and at night.

Modalities:
Aggravation from - By cold weather and air, during sleep & rest, by first motion after rest, by getting wet, in rainy weather, when lying on back or right side and at night.
Amelioration from - By warm, dry weather, motion, walking, change of position, rubbing, warm applications and from stretching out limbs.

SILICEA

This is excellent homoeopathic remedy which is suited to the person who is having diseases of bones, caries and necrosis as a result of Imperfect assimilation and defective nutrition. Person is faint-hearted, anxious and nervous with sensitivity to all impressions.
Indications:

- Stiffness of nape of neck with occipital headache which spreads over head and settled to eyes.

- Weakness of spine with pain in coccyx. Irritation in spine due to injuries to spine.

- Useful for Potts' disease and other diseases of bones of spine.

- Indicated for sciatica, where pain extends from back to hips, legs and feet.
- Cramp in calves and soles with loss of power in legs.

Modalities:
Aggravation from - In morning, from washing, during menses, uncovering the affected part, lying down, in damp, in left side, in cold and in new moon.
Amelioration from - warmth, wrapping up head, in summer and in wet or humid weather.

SULPHUR

It is a great anti-psoric homoeopathic remedy suited for the person which is prone to get various skin affections. It helps to arouse the reactionary powers of the person.
Indications:

- Stiffness of nape with drawing and burning pain between the shoulders.
- Cracking in vertebrae with sensation as if vertebrae glided over each other.
- Sharp and rheumatic pain in left shoulder with heaviness and paretic feeling.
- Rheumatic gout with drawing and tearing pains in arms and hands.

Modalities:

Aggravation from- By rest, when standing, warmth in bed, washing, bathing, in morning, at 11 am, in night and from alcoholic stimulants.

Amelioration from- By dry, warm weather, lying on right side and from drawing up affected limbs.

SYMPHYTUM

An excellent remedy for injuries of bone and cartilages. A great remedy in non-union of fractures.

Indication:

- It helps to heal the fractured bones due to trauma.
- Symphytum may be considered the orthopædic specific of herbal medicine. Pain in back from a fall, from sexual excess. Pott's disease from fall on back.
- Helps to recover the soft parts of bone from the bruised soreness, When the bone or periosteum has been injured.
- Much used remedy among herbalists for caries of spine and other bones.

Modalities:

Aggravation from- By touch or pressure, while walking.

Amelioration from – By warmth.

LESSER KNOWN HOMOEOPATHIC REMEDY FOR SPINAL DISORDERS

BAMBUSA ARUNDINACEA

Bambusa arundinacea is a species of bamboo, of which proving was conducted by 'Bernd Schuster', conducted in 1997. It is em-erging as an important homeopathic remedy for Spine problems.

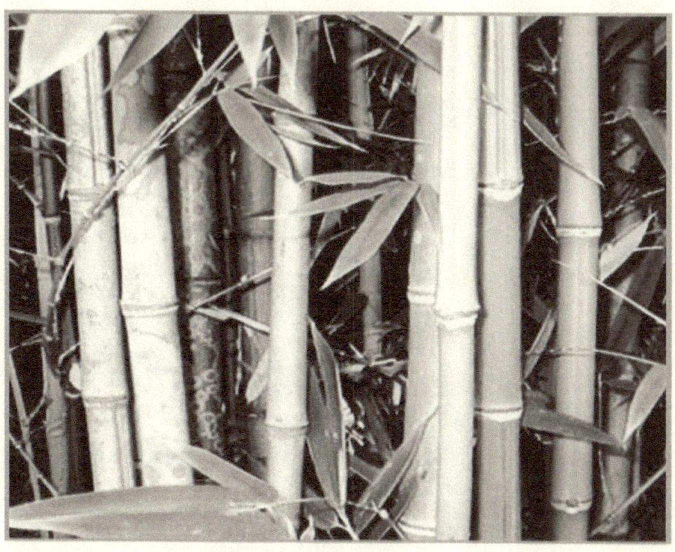

Figure 10.2: Bambusa arundinacea

The homoeopathic preparation of bambusa is prepared by the tincture of bam-boo shoots and contains phyto-oestra-gens and is high in silica. Since ancient times, Bamboo has been used medicinally for cancer, leprosy, tuberculosis, menstrual problems and disorders of the spine.

Indications:

- Great homoeopathic remedy for ankylosing spondylitis. There is painful stiffness of neck; patient often wants to support the neck by rest-ing their chin on their hands.

- There is always a feeling or sensation of stiffness in the spine and body. The stiffness affects primarily the spine and joints near the axis of the body like at shoulders and hips.

- The feeling of stiffness is like of a wood which is very painful, profound and prolonged.

- There is feeling of heaviness like a weight which is felt in the bones, the joints and the muscles.

Modalities:

Aggravation from - By rest and cold, night in bed, or sleep, worse from cold, or cold weather, before and during periods.

Amelioration from - By warmth, applied heat like a hot shower, or bath, or heat pad.

Note: Writer have got very good results from Calcarea Flouricum, Guiacum and Conium for cervical spondylosis, and from Rhus Tox, Kali Carb, Hypericum and Arnica in high potency for Lumbar Spondylosis and Backache.

CHAPTER 11

HOMOEOPATHIC REPERTORY

11.1 Boericke's Repertory

NECK

Burning -- Guaco.

Cracking of cervical vertebrae, on motion --
Aloe, *Cocc.*, *Nat. c.*, Niccol., Ol. an., Thuja.

Emaciation -- Nat. m.

Eruption -- Anac., Clem., Lyc., Nat. m., Petrol., *Sep.*

Fullness, must loosen collar -- *Amyl*, Fel
tauri, *Glon., Lach.*, Pyr., Sep.

Itching -- Ant. c.

Muscles, cervical

Contraction, rigidity -- *Cic.*, Cim., Nicot., *Strych.*

Shooting -- Sul. ac.

Twitching -- Agar.

Muscles, sternocleidomastoid -- *Gels.*, Rhod., Tarax.,
Trifol.

NAPE of the neck

PAINS -- *Acon.*, Ćsc., Am. c., *Bell.*, Chin. ars., *Cim.*, Col., Fel tauri, Ferr. picr., *Gels.*, Graph., Hyper., Jugl. c., Lach., Lyc., Myr., *Nat. chotein*, Nat. s., Paris, Ver. a., Vib. op., X-ray, Zinc. v.

Aching -- Adon. v., Ćsc., Angust., Bapt.,
Caust., *Con., Gels., Guaiac., Paris*, Radium, Ver. v., Ver. v., Zinc. m.
Dislocated, bruised feeling -- Bell., Caust.,
Fagop., *Lachnanth.*
Rheumatic -- Acon, *Bry.*, Calc. p., Caust., *Cim.*,
Colch., *Dulc.*, *Guaiac.*, Iod., Kali iod., *Lachnanth.*, Petrol., Puls., Radium, Rhod., *Rhus t.*, Sang., Stallar., *Sticta.*
Tearing, shooting, stitching -- *Acon.*, Asar., Bad., Bar. c., Bell., *Berb. v., Bry.*, Chin. ars., Colch., Ferr. picr., *Mag. p.*, Nux v., *Strych.*, Xanth.
Tension -- Con., Sep., Sul., Tub.
Tensive numbness -- Plat.

Stiffness -- *Acon.*, Ant. t., *Bell.*, *Bry.*, Calc. c., Calc. *caust.*, Calc. p., Caust., Cham., Chel., *Cim.*, Cocc., Colch., *Dulc.*, Ferr. p., Gels., Guaiac., Hyper., Jugl. c., Kali c., Lac c., *Lachnanth.*, Lyc., Mag. c., Med., Menthol., *Merc. i. r.*, Nicot., Nit. ac., Nux v., Pampin., Petrol., Phos., Phyt., *Puls.*, Radium, Rhodium, Rhod., Rhus v., Sep., Stellar., *Sticta*, Sul., Trifol., Vinca m., X-ray.
Swelling -- Calc. c., Iod., Lyc., Phos., Sil.
Tenderness -- Amyl., *Bry.*, Cim., Kali perm., *Lach.*, Tarax.
Weakness, unable to hold head up -- *Abrot.*, Ćth., Colch., Fagop., Kali c., Sil.

Wryneck (torticollis) -- *Acon.*, Agar., Atrop., *Bell., Bry., Cim., Colch.*, Guaiac., Hyos., Ign., *Lachnanth.*, Lyc., Mag. p., Myg., Nux v., Strych., Thuja.

BACK

Bent, arch-like, opisthotonos -- Angust., Cic., Nat. s., *Nicot.*, Op., Phyt., *Strych.*
Burning -- *Alum., Ars.*, Aur. mur., Berb. v., Calc. fl., Carbo an., HeIod., *Helon.*, Kali p., Lyc., Med., Nit. ac., *Phos., Picr. ac.*, Sep., Tereb., Ustil., Xerophyl.
Scapulć, between -- Glon, *Lyc., Phos.*, Sul.
Spots, in small -- Agar., *Phos.*, Ran. b., Sul.
Coldness -- *Abies c.*, Acon., Ars., Benz. ac., *Gels.*, Gins., Quass., Raph., Sep., *Strych.*, Ver. a.
scapulć, between -- *Abies c., Am. m.*, HeIod., *Lachnanth.*, Sep.
Curvature (scoliosis) -- Bar. c., *Cal. c.*, Phos. ac., Phos., *Sil.*, Sul.
Eruption -- Sep.
Lameness, stiffness -- Abrot., Acon., Ćsc., Agar., Am. m., Bell., *Berb. v., Bry.*, Calc. c., Camph. monobr., *Caust., Cim., Cupr. ars.*, Diosc., Dulc., Gettysburg Water, Gins., *Helon.*, Hyper., *Kali c.*, Kali p., Kal., Lachnanth., Led., Lyc., Nicot., Physost., *Phyt., Rhus t.*, Ruta, Sarcol. ac., *Sep.*, Spong., Staph., *Strych.*, Sul. ac., *Sul.*, Zing.
Numbness -- *Acon., Berb. v.*, Calc. p., *Ox. ac.*, Oxytr., Sec., Sil.

PAIN - Abrot., *Acon., Ćsc., Agar.*, Alum., Am. c.,

Angust., *Ant. t.*, Apis, Arg. m., Arg. n., *Arn.*, Bar. c., Bell., *Berb. v., Bry.*, *Calc. c.*, Calc. p., *Can. ind.*, Carb. ac., Caul., *Caust.*, Cham., Chin. s., Cic., *Cim.*, Cinch., *Cob., Cocc.*, Colch., Col., Dulc., *Eup. perf.*, Graph., *Guaco*, Ham., *Helon.*, Homar., Kali bich., *Kali c.*, Kali m., Lach., Lil. t., Lyc., Mag. m., Mag. s., Med., *Merc.*, Mez., Mormord., Nat. c., *Nat. m.*, Nit. ac., *Nux v.*, Ox. ac., Paraf., Petrol., Phos. ac., *Picr. ac.*, Puls., Radium, Ran. ac., Rhod., *Rhus t.*, Ruta, *Sab.*, Sang., Sarrac., Scolop., Sec., Selen., *Sep.*, Sil., Staph., *Stellar.*, Strych., *Sul.*, Tar. h., *Tellur.*, Ther., Triost., *Upas, Variol.*, Wyeth., Xerophyl., *Zinc. m.*

Aching as if it would break and give out -- *Ćsc.*, Ćth., Am. m., *Bell.*, Can. ind., Cham., *Chel.*, Dulc., *Eup. perf.*, Eupion, Graph., Ham., Kali bich., *Kal.*, Kreos., *Nat. m.*, Ol. an., Ova t., *Phos.*, Plat., *Puls., Rhus t., Sarcol. ac.*, Sanic., Senega, Sil., *Trill.*

Aching, dull, constant (backache) -- *Abies n., Ćsc., Agar.*, Aloe, Am. m., *Ant. t.*, Apoc., Arg. m., Arg. n., *Arn.*, Bapt., Bellis, *Berb. v.*, But. ac., *Calc. c., Calc. fl.*, Canth., *Cim., Cob.*, Coccinel., *Cocc.*, Colch., Con., Conv., Cupr. ars., *Dulc.*, Euonym., Eupion, Ferr. p., Gels., Glycerin, *Helon.*, Hyper., Inula, Ipomśa, Kali c., Kali iod., *Kal.*, Kreos., Lach., Lith. benz., Lycoper., *Lyc.*, Morph., *Nat. m., Nux v.*, Ol. an., *Ol. j. as., Ox. ac.*, Pall., Petrol., Phos. ac., *Phyt.*, Picr. ac., Piscidia., *Pulex, Puls., Radium, Rhus t.*, Ruta, *Sabal*, Sab., Senec., *Sep.*, Solan. lyc., Solid., *Staph., Still., Sul.*, Symphyt., *Tereb.*, Upas, *Vib. op.*, Viscum, Zinc. m.

Scapulć, Between -- *Acon.*, Apomorph., Asclep. t., Bar. c., *Calc. c.*, Can. ind., Con., Guaco, Guaiac., Jugl. c., Kali c., Med., *Pod.*, Radium, *Rhus t.*, Sep., Sul., Zinc. m.

Bruised -- *Acon.*, Ćsc., Agar., Ant. t., *Arn.*, Bar. c., *Berb. v.*, Bry., Cina, *Dulc.*, Gins., Graph., *Ham.*, Mag. s., *Merc.*, Nat. m., *Nux v.*, Phos. ac., Phyt., *Rhus t., Ruta,*Sil., Sul., Tellur.
Crampy -- *Bell.*, Cim., Cinch., *Col.*, Graph., Iris., Mag. p., Ova t., Sep.
Digging, cutting -- Sep.
Drawing -- Anac., Carbo v., *Caust., Kali c.*, Lyc., Nux v., Rhus t., *Sab.*, Sul.
Falling apart sensation, involving small of back, Sacroiliac synchondroses; relieved by bandaging tightly -- Trill.
Heaviness, dragging, weight -- Ćsc., *Aloe, Am. m.*, Anac., Ant. c., Benz. ac., *Berb. v.*, Bov., Colch., *Eup. purp.*, *Helon.*, Hydr., Kali c., *Kreos.*, *Lil. t.*, Nat. s., Picr. ac., *Sep.*
Lancinating, drawing, tearing -- Alum., Asclep. t., *Berb. v.*, Colch., Col., Kali m., Lyc., Mimosa, Nux v., *Scolop.*, Sep., Sil., Stellar., *Strych.*

Extends

Down thighs, legs -- *Ćsc.*, Aur. mur., Bapt., *Berb. v.*, Carb. ac., Cocc., *Col.*, Cur., Ham., *Helon.*, Kali c., Kali m., Lac c., *Ox. ac.*, Phyt., *Scolop., Stellar.*, Tellur., Xerophyl.
Pelvis [to] -- *Arg. n.*, Aur. mur., Berb. v., Cham., *Cim.*, Eupion, Ham., Sil., *Variol.*, Viscum.
Pubes [to] -- *Sab.*, Vib. op., Xanth.
Upwards -- Aspar., *Gels.*

Paralytic -- Cocc., Kali p., Nat. m., Sil.
Pressing, plug-like -- *Ćsc., Agar., Anac.*, Aur. mur., Benz. ac., *Berb. v.*, Colch., Hyper., Nat. m., *Nux v.*, Sep., Tellur.
Sensitiveness extreme of sacrum -- Lob. infl.
Stitching, piercing, pricking -- Agar., Aloe, Alum., Apis., *Berb. v., Bry.*, Guaiac., Hyper., *Kali c., Merc.*, Nat. s., Sul., Tellur., Ther.

MODALITIES

AGGRAVATION

Emission [after] -- Cob.
Masturbation [after] -- Nux v., Phos. ac., Staph.
Night [At] -- Aloe, Calc. c., Lyc., *Merc.*, Mez., Nat. m., *Staph.*, Viscum.
Cold exposure [From] -- Acon., *Bry., Rhod.*, Sul.
Damp exposure [From] -- Dulc., Phyt., *Rhus t.*
Eating [From] -- Kali c.
Exertion [From] -- Agar., *Berb. v.*, Cocc., Hyper., Kali c., Kali p., Ox. ac., Sul.
Jar; touch [From] -- *Acon.*, Berb. v., *Bry.*, Kali bich., *Lob. infl.*, Mez., Sil., *Tellur.*
Lying down [From] -- Bell., *Berb. v.*, Niccol. s., Nux v., Rhus t.
Motion; beginning [From] -- Lac c., *Rhus t.*
Motion; walking [From] -- *Ćsc.*, Aloe, *Ant. t.*, Bell., *Bry., Caust.*, Chel., Cinch., *Colch.*, Kali bich., *Kali c.*, Mez., *Nux v.*, Ox. ac., Paraf., Petrol., Phyt. Ran. ac., Sep., *Sul.*
Resting; sitting [From] -- *Agar.*, Alum., Ant. t., Bell., *Berb. v.*, Can ind., Cob., Ferr. mur., Kali p., Kreos., *Lac c.*, Merc., Nux v., Puls., *Rhus t.*, Sep., Sul., *Zinc. m.*
Standing [From] -- *Ćsc.*, Bell., Nux v., Sarcol. ac., Sep.
Stooping [From] -- *Ćsc.*, Berb. v., Diosc., Guaco, Tellur.
Warmth [From] -- *Kali s.*, Puls., Sul.
Morning [In] -- Agar., *Berb. v.*, Bry., Conv., Kali c., Nat. m., Nux v., Petrol., Phyt., Ruta, Selen., *Staph.*
Rising from seat [When] -- Ćsc., Arg. n., *Berb. v., Caust.*, Kali p., *Lach.*, Sil., Sul., Tellur.

AMELIORATION

Rising [After] -- Kali c., Ruta, Staph.
Bending backward [From] -- Rhus t.
Bending forward [From] -- Lob. infl.
Emission [From] -- Zinc. m.
Lying [From] -- Acet. ac.
Abdomen [on]
Back [on] -- Ćsc., *Cob.*, Gnaph., Nat. m., Rhus t., Ruta.
Something hard, or firm support [on] -- Eupion, *Nat. m., Rhus t.*, Sep.
Lying, sitting [From] -- Sep.
Motion, walking [From] -- Arg. n., Bell., Caust., *Cob.*, Ferr. mur., *Helon.*, Kali m., Kreos., Merc., *Puls.*, Radium, *Rhus t.*, Sep., Staph., *Sul., Zinc. m.*
Rest [From] -- *Ćsc.*, Colch., Nux v., Sil.
Sitting [From] -- Bell.
Standing [From] -- Arg. n., Caust., Sul.
Urination [From] -- *Lyc.*, Med.
WEAKNESS of back -- Abrot., *Ćsc. gl., Ćsc.*, Alum., Ant. t., Arn., Berb. v., But. ac., *Calc. c., Calc. p., Cinch., Cocc.,*Glycerin, Graph., Guaco, *Helon.*, Ign., Irid., Jacar., *Kali c.*, Merc., Nat. m., Nux v., Ox. ac., Petrol., Phos. ac., Phos., *Picr. ac.*, Pod., *Sarrac., Sep., Sil.*, Staph., *Zinc. m.*

BODY

Bruised, sore feeling, all over -- Abrot., Ampel., Apis, *Arn., Bapt., Bellis*, Caust., Cic., Cim., *Cinch., Eup. perf., Gels.*, Ham., Hep., Iberis, Lil. t., *Mang. ac.*, Med., Morph., Nux m., *Phyt.*, Psor., *Pyr., Radium, Rhus* *t., Ruta,*Sarcol. ac., Solan. lyc., Staph., Tellur., *Thuja,*Wyeth.

Burning, in various parts -- Acon., *Agar.*, Apis, *Ars., Canth.*, Caps., *Carbo an.*, Phos. ac., *Phos.*, Sul.

Coldness -- Acon., *Ćth.*, Ant. t., Ars., Atham., *Bar. m., Bor. ac.*, Cadm. s., *Camph.*, Camph. monobr., *Chloral.*, Cupr., *Helod., Jatropha*, Lachnanth., Luffa, *Sec.*, Tab., *Ver. a.*, Zinc. m.

Constriction, as if caged -- Cact., Med.

Numbness -- *Acon.*, Ars., Cic., Con., *Ox. ac., Phos.*, Plumb. m., *Sec.*

Swelling -- *Apis*, Doryph., Frag.

Trembling -- *Agar.*, Cod., *Con., Gels.*, Hyos., Iberis, Lonic., *Myg.*, Phos., Sarcol. ac.

COCCYX

Burning on touch -- Carbo an.

Itching -- Bov., Graph.

Neuralgia, worse rising from sitting posture -- Lach.

Numbness -- Plat.

Pain (coccygodynia) -- Ant. t., Arn., *Bell., Bry., Calc. caust.*, Castorea, *Caust., Cic., Cim.*, Cistus, Con., *Ferr. p.*, Fluor. ac., *Graph., Hyper.*, Kali bich., Kali c., Kali iod., *Kreos.*, Lac c., *Lach.*, Lobel. infl., Mag. c., *Mag. p., Merc., Paris*, Petrol., Phos., *Rhus t.*, Sil., *Tar. h.*, Tetradym., Xanth., Zinc. m.

Bruised -- Am. m., *Arn.*, Caust., Ruta, Sul.

From injury -- Hyper.

Dragging, drawing -- *Ant. t., Caust.*, Graph., Kreos.

Tearing, lancinating -- *Bell.*, Canth., *Cic.*, Kali bich., *Mag. p.*, Merc.

Ulcer -- Pćonia.

LOINS

LUMBAGO -- *Acon.*, Act. sp., *Ćsc.*, Agar., *Aloe, Ant. t., Arn.*, Bell., *Berb. v., Bry., Calc. fl., Calc. p., Carb. ac.*, Carbon. s., *Caul., Cham.*, Chel., *Cim.*, Cina, Colch., Col., Diosc., *Dulc., Eup. perf.*, Ferr. m., *Gins., Gnaph.*, Guaiac., Hydr., *Hymosa*, Ipomśa, Kali bich., *Kali c.*, Kali iod., Kali ox., Lathyr., Led., Lith. benz., Lyc., *Macrot.*, Merc. s., Nat. m., *Nux v.*, Pampin., Picr. ac., Phyt., Puls., Radium, Rham. c., Rhod., *Rhus t.*, Ruta, *Sabal*, Senec., Sep., Spiranth., *Sul.*, Tereb., Vib. op.

Alternates, with headache, piles -- Aloe.

Aggravation [with]

Open air [in] -- Agar.

Beginning to move [on] -- Anac., Con., Glycerin, *Rhus t.*

Relieved by continued motion -- Calc. fl., *Rhus t.*

Exertion [on]; during day; while sitting -- Agar.

Lying down [on] -- Bell., Murex.

Chronic tendency [with] -- Ćsc., Berb. v., *Calc. fl., Rhus t.*, Sil.

Masturbatic origin [with]; sexual weakness -- Nux v.

Numbness [with], in lower part of back, weight in pelvis -- Gnaph.

Relief [with]

Lying down [from] -- Euonym., Sep.

Slow walking [from] -- Ferr. m.

Retching, cold, clammy sweat [with], from least motion -- Lathyr.

Sciatica [with] -- *Rhus t.*

(Normal – 1, *Italic – 2*)

11.2 Kent's Repertory

BACK

ABSCESS: Asaf., *hep.*, iod., lach., mez., *ph-ac., sil.*, staph., *sulph., tarent-c.*
Cervical region: *Lach., lyc., petr.*, ph-ac., psor., sec., *sil., tarent-c.*
old cicatrices: Sil.
Lumbar region: *Calc-p.*
psoas: Ars., *cupr., ph-ac., sil.*, staph., symph., syph.

BIFIDA: Arn., ars., asaf., bar-c., calc-p., *calc-s., calc.*, carb-v., dulc., graph., hep., lach., lyc., merc., mez., nit-ac., phos., *psor.*, ruta., **Sil.**, staph., sulph.
CARIES of spine (CURVATURE of spine): *Bar-m.*, **Calc-f.**, *calc-p.*, **Calc-s., Calc.**, carb-s., *carb-v., con., lyc.*, **Merc-c.**, *merc.*, op., **Ph-ac.**, *phos.*, psor., *puls.*, **Sil., Sulph**., tarent., thuj.
lies on back with knees drawn up: **Merc-c.**
pain in: *Aesc.*, **Lyc., Sil.**
Cervical: *Calc., phos., syph.*
Dorsal: Bar-c., *bufo., calc-s., calc., con., lyc.*, plb., *puls., rhus t., sil., sulph., syph.*, thuj.
lumbar vertebræ: *Sil.*

COLDNESS (including Chill):
Cervical region: *Calc.*, cann-i., carb-s., chel., chr-ac., *dulc.*, fl-ac., ir-foe., kali-chl., laur., lyc., nat-s., op., ran-s., **Sil.**, *spong.*, zinc.
Dorsal region: Agar., croc., *sil.*, spong., thuj.
Lumbar region: Asaf., *camph.*, cann-i., canth., *carb-*

an., carb-s., carb-v., cham., chin., cupr., *dulc.*, **Eup-pur.**, hell., **Lach.**, led., med., nat-m., nux-m., ox-ac., podo., *puls.*, spong., *sulph., sumb.*, tarent.

Sacral region: Arg-m., benz-ac., *dulc.*, hyos., laur., lyc., ox-ac., *puls., sanic.*, stront., sulph.

Spine : Acon., *aesc.*, agar., atro., bol., bry., canth., chlf., coc-c., *crot-c., gels.*, gins., *hyos.*, jug-c., kali-n., lept., meny., merc., *mez.*, mosch., op., ruta., *sanic.*, stry., *sumb.*, tab., thuj., trom.

CONCUSSIONof spine: **Hyper.**

Cervical region: Mez.

CONGESTION, cervical region: Bell., carb-h., **Gels.**, glon., *kali-c.*

CONSTRICTION or band: Alum., anac., arg-n., *cham., cocc., dulc.*, graph., guar., kali-c., mez., nit-ac., rhus-t.

Cervical region: Agar., apis., asar., *bell.*, chel., *glon., lach., nux-m.*, sep.

Lumbar region, as from a tight band: Cina., **Puls.**

CRACKING cervical region: *Agar.*, agn., aloe., anac., aur-m-n., *chel.*, chin., *cocc., nat-c., nicc.*, nit-ac., nux-v., ol-an., *petr.*, puls., raph., spong., stann., *sulph.*, thuj.

Lumbar region, stooping, when: Agar., rhus-t.

walking, while: **Zinc.**

extending to anus: Sulph.

Spine, on moving: *Agar.*, cocc., kali-bi.

CRAMP: Bell., calc-p., iod., kali-bi., lyc., naja., nux-v., plb.

DISLOCATION in last lumbar vertebra, sensation of: Sanic.

EMACIATION: Tab.

Cervical region: *Calc.*, iod., *lyc.*, **Nat-m.**, *sanic., sars.*

Dorsal region, scapular muscles: Plb.
Lumbar region: Plb., sel.
EXOSTOSES on sacrum: Rhus-t.
INJURIES of the
spine: *Apis., arn., calc., con.*, **Hyper.**, *led.*, **Nat-s.**, *nit-ac., rhus-t., ruta., sil., thuj.*
after, lies on back, jerking head backward: *Hyper.*
lifting, from: **Calc., Rhus-t.**
shock of spine: *Arn., hyper., nit-ac.*
Cervical region: Mez.
Lumbar region remains sensitive to jar of walking: *Thuj.*
Coccyx: *Carb-an.*, **Hyper.**, *mez.*, **Sil.**
JERKING in cervical muscles: Aeth., coloc., sep.
NUMBNESS: Acon., *agar.*, berb., *calc-p.*, calc., *cocc.*, cupr-ar., nux-v., ox-ac., phys., sec., sil.
part lain on: Calc.
Cervical region: Berb., cast-eq., *chel.*, dig., hura., merc-i-f., par., *plat.*, rhus-t., tell.
Scapulæ: Anac.
Lumbar region: Acon., ars., Berb., carb-v., *sil.*, spong.
loss of sensation: *Ars.*, bry., con., cupr-ac., kali-n., zinc.
Sacrum: Berb., *calc-p., graph.*, ox-ac., plat., spong.
Coccyx: Berb., **Plat.**
menses, during: Plat.
sitting, while: **Plat.**

OPISTHOTONOS : *Absin.*, acon., agar., amyg., apis., *ars.*, **Bell.**, berb., both., brach., bry., calc-p., *camph., canth.*, carb-an., *cham., chen-a.*, **Cic.**, *cina.*, cor-r., *cupr-ar.*, **Cupr.**, dig., **Hyos.**, hyper., *ign., ip., lach.*, led., med., *morph.*, nat-s., **Nux-v.**, oena., **Op.**, petr., phos., *phyt., plat.*, plb., *rhus-*

t., sec., stann., **Stram., Stry.**, *tab.*, ter., *verat-v., zinc.*
PAIN : Abies-n., acon., **Aesc.**, *aeth., agar.*, ail., aloe., **Alum.**, *alumn.*, am-c., *am-m.*, ambr., anac., anan., *ang.*, ant-c., ant-t., *apis.*, aran., *arg-m., arg-n.*, **Arn.**, ars-i., ars., asaf., asar., *atro.*, aur-m., *aur.*, **Bar-c., Bell.**, *berb., bism., bol.*, bor., brach., brom., **Bry.**, cahin., **Calc-p.**, calc-s., **Calc.**, *camph.*, cann-s., canth., *caps.*, carb-ac., *carb-an.*, **Carb-s.**, *carb-v.*, card-m., *caul., caust., cham., chel.*, chen-a., chin-a., *chin-s.*, chin., chr-ac., cic., *cimic.*, cina., cinnb., clem., cob., coc-c., *cocc., colch., coloc., con.*, cor-r., *crot-h.*, *cub.*, cupr., cycl., dios., *dor.*, dros., dulc., elaps., **Eup-per., Eup-pur.**, *eupho.*, euphr., ferr-ar., ferr-p., *ferr., form.*, gamb., *gels.*, **Graph.**, grat., **Guai.**, gymn., hell., *helon., hep., hydr.*, hyos., *hyper., ign.*, Ind., iod., **Ip.**, *ipom.*, kali-ar., *kali-bi.*, **Kali-c.**, *kali-i., kali-n.*, kali-p., *kali-s., kalm.*, kreos., **Lac-c.**, *lach.*, lact., laur., *led.*, lil-t., lith., *lob.*, **Lyc.**, lyss., mag-c., *mag-m.*, mag-p., mag-s., manc., *med.*, meph., *merc-c., merc., mez.*, **Mur-ac.**, *murx., naja.*, nat-a., *nat-c.*, **Nat-m.**, nat-p., **Nat-s.**, *nit-ac.*, **Nux-m., Nux-v.**, oena., ol-an., ol-j., op., ox-ac., pall., **Par.**, *petr.*, ph-ac., **Phos.**, phys., phyt., plat., *plb.*, podo., **Psor., Puls.**, *ran-b.*, rat., *rhod., rhus-r.*, **Rhus-t.**, *ruta.*, sabad., sabin., *samb.*, sang., sarr., sars., *sec.*, sel., senec., seneg., **Sep., Sil.**, *sol-n.*, spig., spong., stann., *staph.*, stram., *stront.*, *sul-ac.,* **Sulph.**, tarax., tarent., tep., thuj., ust., valer., verat., viol-t., *zinc.*, zing.
daytime: *Camph.*
morning : *Agar.*, all-s., aur., berb., bor., bry., calc-p., canth., cimic., cinnb., dios., dros., equis., eug., eupho., eupi., hep., ign., kali-c., mag-s., naja., *nux-v.*, phyt., podo., puls., *ran-b.*, rhod., ruta., stront., thuj., zinc.

bed, in: Ang., berb., carb-v., eupho., hep., kali-n., mag-s., nat-m., nit-ac., *petr.*, puls., rat., rhod., *ruta.*, staph.
on rising: Am-m., calad., caust., cedr., graph., *hep., lyc., nat-m.*, nit-ac., ran-b., stann., sulph., thuj., verat.
amel.: *Lach.*, nat-c., nat-m., nit-ac.
waking on: Aeth., *agar.*, arg-m., berb., calc-p., cham., chel., grat., kali-bi., lac-c., *lach.*, mag-m., mag-s., myric., nat-m., nit-ac., ptel., ran-b.
forenoon: Ars., *cham.*, equis., *nat-m.*, nat-s., ptel.
10 a.m.: Am-m.
noon: Dios., eupi., rhus-t.
afternoon: Abrot., agar., bov., canth., caust., cham., chel., equis., glon., hyos., mag-c., mag-m., nicc., pall., plb., ptel., rumx., ruta., *sep.*, zing.
evening : Acon., agar., alumn., *ars., calc-p.*, carb-v., cham., chel., cist., cocc., coloc., cupr-ar., ferr-i., gels., kali-ar., kali-n., *kali-s., kalm., lach.*, led., lil-t., *lyc.*, mag-c., mag-m., *naja.*, nat-a., nat-m., nat-s., nit-ac., nux-v., phys., psor., *rhus-t.*, ruta., sarr., *sep.*, sin-n., *sulph.*, ter., thuj., zing.
sunset to sunrise: **Syph.**
night : Acon., agar., aloe., *am-m.*, ang., apis., arg-m., *arg-n., ars., berb.*, bry., calc-s., calc., carb-an., carb-s., carb-v., *cham.*, chel., cinnb., *dulc.*, ferr-ac., ferr-i., ferr-p., *ferr.*, hell., *helon.*, hep., ign., kali-i., kali-n., *kalm., kreos.*, lil-t., lyc., *mag-c.*, mag-m., mag-s., mang., **Merc-c.**, *merc., naja., nat-a., nat-c., nat-m.*, nat-p., *nat-s., nit-ac., nux-v.*, ph-ac., phos., phys., plb., podo., rhod., sars., senec., *sil.*, **Sulph., Syph.**, tab.
between 11 and 12 p.m., violent headache: *Am-m.*
midnight, waking him: *Chin-s.*, nat-c.
before midnight: Kalm.
after: Mag-s.

3 a.m.: **Kali-c.**, kali-n., nat-c.
driving him out of bed: **Kali-c**.
4 a.m.: *Nux-v.*, ruta.
driving him out of bed: *Nux-v.*
acids, after: *Lach.*
air, in cold: Agar., bar-c., *dulc.*, merc., nit-ac., *nux-v., rhus-t.*, sabad., sep.
amel.: **Kali-s.**
draft of, every: *Nux-v.*, verat.
open, amel.: Acon., nux-v., *vib.*
alternating with headache: Aloe., brom., meli.
apyrexia, during: Arn., ars., *calc.*, caps., cham., cina., ign., *nat-m.*, nit-ac., nux-v., petr., samb., sep., sil., spig., stram., thuj., verat.
ascends : Agar., *alum.*, arn., ars., *chin-s.*, clem., *cocc.*, *coloc.*, corn., cycl., dirc., eup-pur., **Gels.**, kalm., kreos., *lach.*, led., mag-m., meny., nat-m., **Nit-ac.**, nux-m., nux-v., ox-ac., *petr.*, phos., *phyt.*, plb., podo., sep., sil., stann., staph., sulph., ust.
constriction of anus, with: *Coloc.*
descends, and: Kali-c.
labor, during: **Gels.**, *petr.*
lying down, after: Mag-m.
sitting, while: Meny.
spreading upwards like a fan: *Lach.*
step, during every: Sep.
stool, during: Phos., podo.
stooping: Arn., *sil.*
twinges up the, better by drawing shoulders back: Cycl.
bending backward agg.: Arg-m., bar-c., *calc-p., calc., chel., cimic.*, con., dios., kali-c., lam., mang., plat., puls., sel., stann.

amel.: Acon., aeth., am-m., bell., cycl., eupi., fl-ac., hura., lach., petr., puls., rhus-t., sabad., sabin., sil.
forward agg.: *Pic-ac.*
amel.: Chel., meny., nat-a., ph-ac., puls., sang., sec., sep., thuj.
breathing, when : Acon., aesc., alum., alumn., *am-m.*, apis., arn., asar., *aur.*, berb., calc., cann-s., carb-an., carb-s., carb-v., cham., chel., cinnb., **Coloc.**, conv., *cop.*, cupr-ar., cupr., dig., dulc., inul., kali-bi., *kali-c.*, kali-n., kali-p., kali-s., kalm., led., lob., merc., mur-ac., nat-a., nat-c., nat-m., nux-v., par., petr., prun-s., *psor.*, ptel., puls., raph., ruta., sabin., sang., sars., seneg., *sep.*, spig., stann., *sulph.*, thuj.
chill, before: **Aesc.**, aran., *ars.*, bry., carb-v.,
daph., *dios., eup-per.*, eup-pur., *ip.*, **Podo.**, rhus-t.
during : Ant-t., apis., *arn., ars., bell.,* **Bol.**, calc., *caps.*, carb-s., carb-v., caust., *cham.*, chin-a., **Chin-s.**, chin., elat., *eup-per.*, gamb., hyos., ign., *ip.*, lach., lact-ac., lyc., mosch., myric., *nat-m.*, **Nux-v.**, phos., podo., *puls.*, sang., sep., sulph., verat., zinc.
extending to occiput and vertex: **Puls.**
coffee agg.: *Cham.*
coition, after: Cann-i., **Nit-ac.**, *sabal.*
cold weather, change to: **Calc-p., Dulc.**, rhod., *rhus-t.*
taking: *Dulc.*, mag-p., nit-ac., sars.
convulsions, with: Acon.
coughing, when : *Acon.*, *am-c.*, arn.,
arund., **Bell., Bry.,**calc-s., *calc., caps.*, carb-an., chin-s., chin., cocc., cor-r., *kali-bi.*, kali-c., kali-n., kreos., *merc., nit-ac.*, ph-ac., phos., puls., rhus-t., rumx., seneg., *sep.*, stram., sulph., tell.
damp weather: **Calc., Dulc.**, *nux-m., phyt., rhod.,* **Rhus-t.,**sep.

descends : Acon., *aeth.*, alum., am-c., chel., cimic., cina., cocc., con., cur., elaps., ferr-s., *glon.*, kali-bi., *kali-c., kalm.*, lil-t., mag-c., mang., merc., nat-m., nat-s., *nux-m.,* nux-v., ox-ac., phys., *phyt., pic-ac.*, podo., psor., rat., sang., sep., thuj., ust., zing.
during labor: *Nux-v.*
dinner, after: Agar., cob., indg., phel., phos., sep., sulph.
drinking, while: Chin.
eating, while: Chin., coc-c.
after: Agar., ant-t., bry., cham., cina., *daph., kali-c.*
amel.: Kali-n.
emissions, after: Ant-c., cob., kali-br., ph-ac., sars., *staph.*
eructation amel.: *Sep.*
exertion, from: *Agar.*, asaf., calc-p., calc., ox-ac., ruta., *stry.*, sulph.
amel.: Ruta., *sep.*
fasting, when: Kali-n.

PAIN, motion,
amel. by gentle: Bell., *calc-f.*, ferr., *kali-p.*, **Puls.**
move, beginning to: Bry., **Caps.**, *carb-v.*, caust., **Con., Ferr.**, *kali-p.*, **Lyc.,** *phos.*, **Puls., Rhus-t.**, sep., sil., tab., zinc.
compelling to, constantly in bed: Phos., *puls.*, **Rhus-t.**
compelled to, no relief: *Lact.*, **Puls.**
music, from: Ambr.
noise agg.: Ars., **Ther.**
running water: *Lyss.*
nursing, while: Cham., crot-t., puls., **Sil.**
paralytic: *Cocc.*, kalm., nat-m., ran-s., *sabin.*, zinc.
paroxysmal: Asaf., kalm., lyss., nat-c., pall., phos.
periodical: *Ars., chin-s.*, kali-s.

perspiration, during: Carb-v., **Merc.**
pressure: Acon., aesc., agar., ang., arn., canth., chel., chin-s., cocc., *colch.*, coloc., crot-t., *hep.*, lach., phos., plat., plb., ruta., sulph., thuj., verb.
amel.: Aur., camph., carb-ac., cimic., *dulc.*, fl-ac., **Kali-c.**, led., mag-m., *nat-m.*, ph-ac., plb., *rhus-t.*, ruta., **Sep.**, verat., vib.
pulling agg.: Dios.
pulsating: Am-c., sil.
raising arms, on: *Graph.*
thigh, while sitting: Agar.
reaching up: **Rhus-t.**
reading, while: Nat-c.
rheumatic : Acon., ambr., anac., ant-t., *ars.*, asar., aspar., aur., bapt., bar-c., bell., **Bry.**, *calc-p., calc.*, calen., *carb-v.*, cham., *chel.*, **Cimic.**, *colch.*, com., *corn.*, cycl., dros., *dulc., ferr.*, graph., *guai.*, *hep., kali-bi., kali-i.*, lach., lyc., *lycps., med.*, mez., **Nux-v.**, ol-an., petr., *phyt., puls.*, ran-b., **Rhod., Rhus-t.**, *ruta., sang.*, squil., stram., *sulph.*, teucr., ust., valer., verat., zinc.
riding in a carriage: Calc., carb-ac., fl-ac., kali-c., lac-c., **Nux-m.**, *petr.*, sep., sulph., ust.
on horseback: Ars.
rising from sitting: Aesc., **Agar.**, alum., ant-c., apis., aran., arg-n., *ars.*, **Berb.**, bry., *calc-s., calc.*, cann-i., *canth.*, carb-an., **Caust.**, con., ferr-p., ferr., iris., *kali-bi.*, kali-p., *led.*, lyc., **Merc.**, merl., petr., **Phos.**, ptel., **Puls.**, rhod., **Rhus-t.**, ruta., sep., *sil., staph.*, **Sulph.**, tab., tell., thuj., tus-p., *zinc.*
long, almost impossible: *Aesc., agar.*, am-c., *bell., berb., calc., phos.*, **Puls., Rhus-t**.
stooping: *Aesc.*, agar., am-m., *berb.*, bism., chel., *eupi.*, kali-

bi., lach., *lyc.*, med., mur-ac., *nat-m.*, ph-ac., *phos.*, **Puls.**, *rhus-t.*, sars., *sil., sulph.*, verat., *zinc.*

stooping, prolonged: *Nat-m.*, **Puls.**

rubbing amel.: Aeth., kali-n., lach., lil-t., nat-s., **Phos.**, plb., puls., thuj.

sewing, while: Iris., sec.

sexual excesses: Ars., calc., carb-v., *chin., nat-m., nat-p.*, **Nux-v., Ph-ac.**, *phos., puls., sep.*, **Staph.**, *sulph.*

sitting, while : **Agar.**, aloe., am-m., ambr., *ant-t.*, apis., **Arg-m.**, arg-n., asaf., asar., aspar., bar-c., *berb.*, bor., *bry.*, calc-f., *calc., cann-i.*, carb-an., carb-s., *carb-v., caust.*, cham., chin-s., chin., cimx., cist., cob., cocc., coff., con., cycl., dros., dulc., equis., euphr., ferr-p., ferr., fl-ac., helon., hep., hura., hyos., kali-bi., *kali-c.*, kali-i., kali-n., kali-p., kali-s., *lach., led., lyc.*, mag-c., mag-m., meny., merc., mur-ac., nat-a., nat-c., nat-m., nat-p., *nat-s., nux-v.*, ol-an., ox-ac., pall., par., *ph-ac.*, phel., *phos.*, pic-ac., podo., *prun-s., puls., rhod.*, **Rhus-t.**, *ruta.*, sabad., **Sep.**, sil., spong., stann., *sulph.*, tab., ter., *thuj.*, ust., **Valer., Zinc.**

amel.: Aeth., bor., caust., mag-c., meny., mur-ac., plb., sars., staph.

dyspnœa, with: Lyc.

erect: **Kali-c.**, spong., **Sulph.**

bent: Chel., chin-s., kali-i., laur., nat-c., phos., ran-b., sec., sep., thuj.

has to sit: **Kali-c., Sulph.**

long, after: Aloe., asaf., berb., *calc., cupr-ar., led.*, lith., *ph-ac., phos.*, **Puls.**, *rhod., rhus-t.*, thuj., valer.

sleep, during: *Am-m.*, ars., kalm., lach., puls., zinc.

ongoing to: Mag-m.

sound, after falling into: *Am-m.*, kalm., *lach.*

sneezing when: Arn., arund., *sulph.*

before: Anag.
speaking, when: Cocc.
standing, while : *Agar.*, agn., asar., berb., *bry., calc.*, cann-i., caps., cocc., coff., *con.*, hep., ign., Ind., kali-bi., kali-c., kali-p., *kali-s.*, lil-t., lith., lyc., meny., merc., mur-ac., nit-ac., petr., *ph-ac., phos.*, plan., plb., podo., puls.,
rumx., *ruta., sep.*, spong., **Sulph.**, thuj., tus-p., **Valer.**, verat., zinc.
amel.: *Arg-n., bell.*, mur-ac.
erect almost impossible after sitting: *Thuj.*
leaning sideways, while: Thuj.
stepping, when: Acon., carb-ac., carb-an., sep., spong., *sulph., ther., thuj.*
false: Podo., *sep., sulph., ther., thuj.*
stool, before: Bapt., cic., kali-n., *nux-v.*, petr., puls.
during: Apis., *ars.*, carb-an., colch., coloc., cupr., cycl., *dulc.*, ferr-ar., ferr., kali-i., *lyc.*, manc., nicc., nux-v., phos., *podo., puls.*, rheum., squil., stront., sulph., tab., zing.
after: Aesc., aloe., alum., asaf., berb., caps., colch., dig., dros., *ferr.*, mag-m., nat-m., podo., *puls.*, rheum., tab.
amel.: Nux-v., ox-ac., puls.
urging to: Zing.
stooping, when : *Aesc.*, **Agar.**, *alum.*, arn., bor., bov., *bry.*, bufo., caps., *carb-v., cham., chel.*, clem., *cocc.*, con., corn., daph., dig., dios., *dulc.*, hep., hura., hyos., kali-bi., *kali-c.*, kali-n., lyc., mang., meny., nat-m., nux-v., ol-an., par., pic-ac., plb., puls., rhod., *rhus-t.*, ruta., sabin., sars., **Sep.**, *sil.*, stront., sul-ac., *sulph.*, tell., thuj., verat., *zinc.*
prolonged, from: **Nat-m.**
straightening up the back: Aeth., agar., bufo., calc., *cann-i.*, carb-ac., chel., *kali-bi.*, kali-c., lach., nat-c., *nat-m.*, nux-v., *psor., sep., sulph., thuj.*

amel.: Bov., laur.
stretching: Calc., mag-c.
struck with a hammer, as if: **Sep.**
supper, after: Sulph.
swallowing, on: *Caust.*, *kali-c.*, raph., *rhus-t.*
talking prevented: Cann-i.
throwing shoulders backward amel.: Cycl.
thunderstorm, during agg.: Agar., rhod.
turning, when: *Agar.*, am-m., bov., *bry.*, dios., hep., kali-bi., merc., *nux-v., sanic.*, sars., sep., sil., thuj., verat.
in bed, when: Acon., *bry.*, calad., hep., ign., kali-bi., kali-n., mag-m., merc., nat-c., *nux-v.*, sep., *staph.*, sulph., zinc.
amel.: Nat-m.
compels: Phos., **Rhus-t.**
must sit up to turn over: Kali-p., **Nux-v.**
head agg.: *Caust.*, lachn., sanic.
to left, pain in trapezius: Bry.
suddenly: Mag-m.
ulcerative pain in back: Kreos., puls.
urinate, with the desire to: Clem., eupi., *lach.*, nat-s.
urinating, before: Graph., *lyc.*
during: *Ant-c., ip., kali-bi.,* phos., *sulph.*
after: Caust., *syph.*
amel.: **Lyc.**, med.
urine, on retaining: Arn., con., *nat-s.*, rhus-t.
vexation, after: Nux-v.
waking, on: Abrot., aesc., arg-m., berb., calc-p., chel., hep., *lach.*, mag-m., mag-s., myric., ptel., puls., rhod.

STIFFNESS : Acon., aesc., *agar., alum., am-m., anac.*, anan., *ang., apis.*, arg-n., *ars.*, aur-m., aur., *bapt., bar-c., bell., benz-ac.*, **Berb.**, *bol., bry., calc-*

s., calc., carb-an., carb-s., *carb-v., carl.,* **Caust.,** cedr., *chel., cic.,* **Cimic.,** cocc., con., cop., cupr-ar., cupr., dig., gins., *guai., helon.,* hydr., *ign.,* Ind., iris., jac., *kali-ar.,* kali-bi., *kali-c., kali-p., kali-s., lach.,* **Led.,** *lyc., manc.,* med., nat-a., nat-m., nat-s., *nit-ac.,* **Nux-v.,** ol-an., olnd., op., *petr., phos., phyt., prun-s., puls.,* rheum., **Rhus-t.,** rhus-v., **Sep., Sil.,** *staph., stram., stry.,* sul-ac., **Sulph.,** tab., *thuj.,* tub., verat., zinc., zing.

STRAINING, easy: Bor., **Calc., Graph., Lyc.,** *nux-v.,* ph-ac., **Rhus-t.,** sang., *sep.*

TENSION : Aeth., *agar.,* am-m., arg-n., *ars.,* bar-c., berb., bry., coloc., con., hep., ign., *lil-t., lyc.,* med., mez., mosch., nat-c., nat-m., ol-an., olnd., *puls.,* rat., sars., sep., *sulph.,* tarax., teucr., thuj., zinc.

Cervical region : Agar., aloe., **Alum.,** am-m., ant-c., *apis.,* aur., *bar-c.,* **Bell.,** berb., bov., *bry.,* calc., camph., carb-an., *carb-s., carb-v., caust., chel.,* **Cic., Cimic.,** cinnb., colch., cupr., dig., dulc., elaps., eupho., *gels.,* glon., graph., *hell.,* hyos., hyper., iod., ip., kali-c., kali-s., *lac-c., lyc., mag-s.,* med., mez., mosch., *nat-c., nat-m., nat-s.,* nicc., nit-ac., *nux-m., ol-an.,* par., *plat.,* plb., psor., *puls., rat., rhod., rhus-t.,* sars., sep., sil., *spong., staph., stram.,* stront., *sulph., thuj.,* verat-v., verat., *zinc.*

Dorsal region: Aur-m., crot-c., lyc., mag-s., *rhus-t., zinc.*

walking amel.: Mag-s.

scapulæ: Alum., *bar-c.,* **Carb-an.,** cic., colch., *coloc.,* con., kali-c., lyc., mag-m., merc-c., merc., *mez.,* mur-ac., nat-c., *nux-v.,* op., *rhus-t.,* sep., sil., sulph., zinc.

Lumbar region : Acon., *agar.,* ambr., aur-m., *bar-c.,* **Berb.,** bov., brom., bry., carb-s., carb-v., *carl.,* caust., *chin.,* clem.,.

coc-c., *colch.*, cycl., lyc., merl., *nat-m.*, nit-ac., *nux-v., phos., puls.*, rheum., sep., sil., *sulph.*, thuj., verat., *zinc.*
Sacrum: *Bar-c.*, berb., caust., puls., sars., *sulph.*, tarax., *zinc.*

TINGLING:
Cervical region: Arund., *carl.*, dulc., lac-c., phos., sabin., *sec.*, spong.
on entering a house: Phos.
Dorsal region, scapulæ: *Anac.*, sil., zinc.
shoulders, between the: Carl., laur., viol-t.
Lumbar region: Acon., ars., arund., bufo-s., canth., crot-t., meny., merc-c., ph-ac., stann., tarax., thuj.
Sacrum: Bor., crot-t., ph-ac., sars.
Spine: **Acon., Agar.**, *ars.*, arund., con., kali-p., *lach.*, nat-c., *sal-ac.*

TREMBLING: Apis., carb-v., cimic., *cocc.*, eup-per., lil-t.
Scapulæ: *Sulph.*
Lumbar region: Benz-ac., berb., cimic., merc., oci.

TUMORS, pediculated bluish as large as a cherry: *Con.*, thuj.
fatty, on neck: **Bar-c.**, calc., *thuj.*
malignant on neck: Calc-p.
sarcoma: *Bar-c.*

TWITCHING: *Agar.*, alum., calc., chel., jatr., kali-bi., merc., mez., morph., mygal., nat-m., petr., phys., spig., stry., sulph., *zinc.*
Cervical region: Aeth., arn., bufo., caust., coloc., mag-m., nat-m., ph-ac., ran-b., sep., sulph.
rest, during: Ph-ac.

tearing, extending into vertex, while walking: Rat.
Dorsal region: Nit-ac., *stry.*
scapulæ: Calc-p., calc., lyc., merc., mez., nat-c., phos., rhus-t., sep., squil., thuj.
Lumbar region: *Agar., alum.*, calc., *coloc.*, con., crot-t., dulc., lach., petr., rat., sumb.
Coccyx: Alum., *cic.*
menses, during: *Cic.*
painful: Alum.

ULCERS: *Cist., merc-c.*
Cervical region: Sil.
Dorsal region, scapulæ: Kali-bi., merc.
Sacrum: *Arg-n., ars.*, crot-h., *paeon., zinc.*
burn like fire: *Ars.*
Coccyx: Paeon.
WARM,sense of warm air steaming up spine into head: *Ars.*

WEAKNESS (tired feeling, in spine) :
Abrot., *aesc.*, aeth., *agar.*, alumn., anan., ant-t., apis., **Ars.**, bar-c., berb., *brach.*, calc-s., **Calc.**, carb-ac., carb-s., carb-v., *casc.*, cast., chin-a., *cic.*, cimic., coloc., cupr-ar., cur., *eup-per., gels.*, gins., **Graph.**, guai., helon., hep., hydr., iris., kali-cy., kali-p., *lach.*, lob., *lyss.*, med., *murx.*, nat-a., **Nat-m.**, nat-p., nit-ac., **Nux-v.**, ol-j., ox-ac., pall., petr., **Ph-ac.**, *phos.*, phys., *pic-ac.*, plb., podo., psor., *puls.*, raph., *rhus-t.*, sarr., **Sel., Sep., Sil.**, sul-ac., **Sulph.**, tell., ther., verat-v., **Zinc.**
Cervical region : Acon., *aesc., agar.*, aloe., ars-m., *cact.*, cimic., **Cocc.**, *gels., glon., kali-c., lach.*, nit-ac., *par.*, petr., phos., pic-

ac., *plat., sil., stann.*, staph., *verat.*, viol-o., *zinc.*
manual labor: *Agar., kali-c., lach.*, nit-ac., *sil.*, verat.
writing, while: **Zinc.**
Dorsal region, scapulæ, amel. stooping: Alumn.
between: *Agar.*, sarr.
leaning on something, amel.: Sarr.
Lumbar region : *Aesc., agar.*, all-s., *alum.*, alumn., am-c., ambr., *arg-n.*, arn., **Ars.**, aur-m., aur., bar-c., *bell.*, benz-ac., **Calc-s., Calc.**, camph., carb-ac., carb-s., carl., chel., cimic., cimx., *cina.*, clem., **Cocc.**, *coloc.*, con., dios., *eup-per., graph., helon., hep.*, hura., hydr., *kali-bi., kali-c.*, kali-cy., kali-i., kali-s., *lach.*, laur., *lec., led.*, lil-t., *lycps.*, lyss., manc., meph., merc-i-f., *merc.*, morph., *mur-ac., murx.*, naja., nat-c., **Nat-m.**, nat-p., *nux-m.*, nux-v., *nym., ox-ac., pall.*, petr., *phos.*, phyt., **Pic-ac.**, plan., *psor.*, ptel., **Puls.**, raph., **Rhus-t.**, *rhus-v.*, rumx., *ruta.*, sabin., sanic., *sec.*, **Sel.**, senec., **Sep.**, *sil.*, sul-ac., sul-i., **Sulph.**, thuj., *zinc.*

WIND, as if blowing between shoulders:
Caust., *hep.*, sulph.
Lumbar region: *Sumb.*

(Normal – 1, *Italic – 2*, **Bold - 3)**

11.3 C.M. Boger's Short Repertory

BACK, SPINE AND CORD

Back, spine and cord : **Agar.**, Ars., Aur., *Bell.*, **Calc-c.**, Chin-s., *Cimi.*, Cocc., Gels., Hyper., Kali-c., *Lach.*, Nat-m., Nat-s., *Nux-v.*, Pho-ac., **Pho.**, *Pic-ac., Rhus-t.*, Sec-c., **Sil.**, *Sul., Zin.*

Back, spine and cord, right: Calc-c., Cic., Flu-ac., *Sul.*, Zin.

Back, spine and cord, right to left: Calc-p., Cocc., Kali-p., Sul., Tell.

Back, spine and cord, left: Dros., Glo., Sil.

Back, spine and cord, left to right: Bell., Cond., Nat-c., Ox-ac.

Back, spine and cord, alternating sides: Agar., Bell., *Berb.*, Calc-p., Kali-bi., Kalm.

Back, spine and cord, alternating sides, with headache: Aco., Alu., Brom., Ign., Melil., Sep.

Back, spine and cord, catching in: Dios.

Back, spine and cord, changing here and there: Berb., Cimi., Kali-bi.

Back, spine and cord, chest, into: Aco., Arn., Bar-c., Berb., *Bry.*, Calc-p., Cam., Kali-c., Kali-n., Laur., Lyc., Merc., Mez., Petr., Plat., Samb., Sars., Sep., Zin.

Back, spine and cord, chest, into, left: Bar-c., *Bry.*, Mez., Plat., Zin.

Back, spine and cord, chest, into, right: Aco., Calc-p., Kali-c., Lyc., Merc., Sep.

Back, spine and cord, upward: Gels., Lach., Lil-t., Nit-ac., Pho., Sul.

Back, spine and cord, blow or sudden shock: Bell., Cic., *Sep.*, Stan.

Back, spine and cord, broken, as if: Arn., *Bell.*, Ham., *Kali-c.*, Lyc., Nat-m., Pho.

Back, spine and cord, burning, heat: Agar., Alu., *Ars.*, Bapt., Carb-an., Kali-bi., *Lyc.*, *Pho.*, Sec-c., Sil., Sul.

Back, spine and cord, burning, heat, spine: Kali-bi.,

Lyc., *Pho.*

Back, spine and cord, burning, upward in: Bapt., Pho.

Back, spine and cord, coldness: Merc., Nux-v., Pul., Sil., Sul., Ver-a.

Back, spine and cord, coldness, down: Canth., Eup-p., Lac-c., Stram.

Back, spine and cord, coldness, spine (interscapular): Agar., *Am-m.*, Arg-n., Caps., Helo., Hyo., Lachn., Med., Petr., *Polyp.*, Rhus-t., Sec-c.

Back, spine and cord, cramp: Caust., *Chin.*

Back, spine and cord, forward, scapular region: Bry., Sul., Zin.

Back, spine and cord, forward, scapular region, left: Sul., Zin.

Back, spine and cord, forward, lumbar region: *Berb.*, Cham., *Kali-c.*, Kre., **Sabi.**

Back, spine and cord, forward, around pelvis: Sabi., Sep., Vib.

Back, spine and cord, motion, agg.: Kali-c.

Back, spine and cord, numbness: Aco., Agar., *Berb.*, Bry., Kali-bi., *Ox-ac.*, Plat., Sep.

Back, spine and cord, plug, lump, etc., as of a: *Arn.*, Berb., *Carb-v.*, Pho.

Back, spine and cord, pressure, agg.: Agar., *Bell., Chin-s.*, Cimi., Pho.

Back, spine and cord, pressure, amel.: Bry., *Dulc.*, **Kali-c.**, *Nat-m.*, Rhus-t., Rut., *Sep.*

Back, spine and cord, sharp, darting, shooting: Kali-c., Nat-m., Ox-ac.

Back, spine and cord, short, as if: Agar., Aur., Hyo., Lyc., Sul.

Back, spine and cord, sitting, agg.: Zin.

Back, spine and cord, spots, agg. in: Agar., *Alu.*, Caust., Chel., Chin., Kali-bi., *Lach.*, Nit-ac., Ox-ac., Pho-ac., *Pho.*, Plb., Rhus-t., Thu., Zin.
Back, spine and cord, stiff: *Berb.*, *Caust.*, Dulc., Kali-c., Led., Nux-v., Pul., Rhus-t., *Sep.*, Sil., *Sul.*
Back, spine and cord, swallowing, agg.: Caust., Kali-c., *Rhus-t.*
Back, spine and cord, throbbing: Bar-c., Bell., Lyc., Nat-m., Pho., Sep., Sil., Thu.
Back, spine and cord, weak: Ars., Bar-c., Calc-c., *Cocc.*, Grap., Kali-c., Nat-m., Nux-v., Pho-ac., Pho., Sele., Sep., Sil., Zin.

SCAPULAR REGION.

Scapular region:
Chin., Dulc., Kali-c., Kre., Merc., Rhus-t., *Sep.*
Scapular region, between:
Am-m., Ars., Calc-c., Calc-p., Helo., Pho.
Scapular region, underneath:
Calc-c., *Gels.*, Merc.

DORSAL REGION.

Dorsal region:
Arn., Ars., *Bell., Calc-c.*, Caust., Chin., *Cocc.*, Gels., Ign., Lyc., *Nat-m., Nux-v.*, Pho., Pic-ac., *Pul., Rhus-t.*, Rut., Sep., Sil., *Sul.*
Dorsal region, curvature:
Aur., Calc-c., Lyc., Merc., *Pul., Sul.*
Dorsal region, emaciated:
Nux-v.
Dorsal region, sensitive, spine:
Agar., Bell., Chin-s., Cimi., Hyper., Ign., Nux-v., Pho.,

Zin.

Dorsal region, stiff:

Caust., Rhus-t.

Dorsal region, weak:

Pic-ac.

Dorsal region, weak, interscapular:

Agar., Alu., *Bur-p.*, Radm-b., Sars.

LUMBAR REGION.

Lumbar region:

Aesc., Alu., *Ant-t.*, Ars., Berb., *Calc-c.*, Caust., Cimi., Kali-c., Nux-m., **Nux-v.**, Pul., **Rhus-t.**, *Sep.*, Sul., Variol.

Lumbar region, to chest:

Berb., Sul.

Lumbar region, chill, starts in:

Gels., Hyo., Lach., *Nat-m.*, Stro., Sul.

Lumbar region, cold:

Bry., Canth., *Eup-p.*, Gels., *Lach.*, Merc-c., Rhus-t., *Sul.*

Lumbar region, forward in:

Berb., Cham., Kali-c., Kre., **Sabi.**

Lumbar region, forward in, around pelvis:

Sabi., Sep., Vib.

Lumbar region, lumbago:

Ant-t., Bell., Kali-bi., Nux-v., Ox-ac., *Rhus-t.*, Sec-c.

Lumbar region, stitches:

Berb., *Bry.*, Coloc., *Kali-c.*, Lyc., Pul.

SACRUM.

Sacrum:

Grap., Hep., Hyper., Rhus-t.

(Normal – 1, *Italic – 2*, **Bold - 3)**

Bibliography

- Orthopedics Quick Review (Opqr): Magic Book of Orthopedics- Seventh edition by Apurv Mehra
- Essential Orthopaedics - fourth edition by J. Maheshwari
- Textbook Of Orthopedics Includes Clinical Examination Methods In Orthopedics – fifth edition by John Ebnezar
- Organon of medicine – by Dr. Samuel Hahnemann
- The Genius of Homoeopathy – by Dr. Stuart Close
- The principles and the art of cure by homoeopathy – By Dr. H. A. Roberts
- Lectures on theory and practice of homoeopathy – Dudgeon

- Principles and practice of homoeopathy – Richard Hughes

- Homoeopathy in Cervical Spondylosis – First edition by Dr. Farokh J. Master

- Boericke's New Manual of Homeopathic Materia Medica with Repertory - Third Revised & Augmented Edition Based on Ninth Edition by William Boericke

- Repertory of the Homoeopathic Materia Medica – J.T. Kent

- Confronting Chronic Pain, A Pain Doctor's Guide to Relief – by Steven H. Richeimer, MD with Kathy Steligo

- Everything You Wanted to Know About the Back, A Consumer's Guide to the Diagnosis and Treatment of Lower Back Pain – by Donald S. Corenman, MD, DC

- Yoga for Back Pain - by Loren Fishman MD, Carol Ardman

- Yoga for a Healthy Lower Back: A Practical Guide to Developing Strength and Relieving Pain - by by Liz Owen, Holly Lebowitz Rossi

- The Back-Pain Relief Diet: The Undiscovered Key to Reducing Inflammation and Eliminating Pain 1st Edition - by Todd Sinett

- http://www.allaboutbackpain.com
- http://www.nlm.nih.gov
- http://www.ct-ortho.com
- http://en.wikipedia.org
- http://www.webmd.com
- http://www.healthcentral.com
- http://www.healthline.com
- https://www.radiologyinfo.org
- https://www.ucsfhealth.org
- https://homeopathyinformation.com
- https://osteoporosis.ca
- http://www.premierortho.com

www.ingramcontent.com/pod-product-compliance
Lightning Source LLC
La Vergne TN
LVHW050408160726
843469LV00041B/996

* 9 7 8 9 3 5 4 5 8 4 4 4 2 *